the women on my couch

MORE STORIES
OF SEX, LOVE AND
PSYCHOTHERAPY

dr. brandy engler

The Women on My Couch
Copyright 2015 © Dr. Brandy Engler

Contents

Intro

I'd always intended to do sex therapy with women. In grad school, I'd fought to host a performance of the *Vagina Monologues* at a conservative college, and I'd written my dissertation on women's libido. I saw myself as a feminist psychologist with a mission to help women claim the power of their sexuality.

When I hung my first shingle in Times Square, to my surprise the only calls that came were from men. Suddenly, I was tasked to treat chronic womanizing and cuckold fetishes and addiction to massage parlors. These guys initially tested my sensibilities, but my job was to help. I'd developed a new compassion for the inner struggles of men and was so inspired by the shift in my worldview that I wrote a memoir called *The Men on My Couch*. Soon after, I became a contributor to *Men's Health* magazine and was even dubbed by *London Times* the "Wall Street Sex Therapist," but I hadn't forgotten my original purpose.

Eventually, I moved to Los Angeles and opened a private practice. In an effort to attract women, I simply changed one word in my advertising. I switched from a specialty of "sex" to "*relationships* and sex." At last, the calls came in.

Women arrived on my couch, and their topics of conversation spanned from love addiction to low libido. There were broken hearts and hot affairs and kinky propositions to decide about. Fresh with the knowledge of men's perspective on sex and relationships, I found myself more challenging to women than I would've been if I didn't have that year with men. Armed with an awareness of the mistakes women make—such as having unrealistic expectations, being passive or critical—and the dire consequences these have on relationships, I chose to hold women accountable: to be self-reflective, to be better lovers, and to rise out of the victim narrative. I was not easy on women, but I remained as compassionate, this time because I could identify with their mistakes. I had to learn many of the same lessons. And even though treating men was difficult for me, therapy with women was much more complicated.

There are no easy answers to the modern sexual dilemmas women face. Contemporary sexuality, with its diversity and liberation, has created a vast gray area—and it is in this space where conflicts and questions arise. What the women on my couch wanted was help navigating their choices: a husband's proposition for a threesome, participation in a new boyfriend's kink—one that half offends and half arouses—the temptation to use sex work to pay off student loan debt, or how to deal with the discovery that marriage is "a constant inconvenience."

Women are making more money, old hierarchies are being upended, and people's sexual tastes are struggling to adapt to what's happening outside the bedroom. Some women are rejecting marriage, children, and even love. And, of course, the good old-fashioned "Sorry, honey, I have a headache" scenario remains the most popular issue showing up in my practice—except often it's the men who have the headache.

My couch was on the frontier of women's sexual issues, of social change playing out in the bedroom. No standardized treatment protocols even existed for the quandaries I was encountering. As such, this is not a prescriptive book full of simple tips, but I do show, in a fly-on-the-wall fashion, what happens in the therapy room, as we steer through a process for making decisions mindfully. Sex is a great tool for personal growth and a window into the self; the unconscious mind speaks and the body betrays our truth. Sex shows us the edges of our ability to be intimate, to speak up, and to have a sturdy sense of self.

California's therapy scene has long been a purveyor of alternative practices. For me, it was the perfect place to explore new treatment ideas for women. Any therapist from New York is heavily influenced by psychoanalysis and other traditional approaches, so when I came to

California and heard words like "healing" or "energy," I thought, *Really? How do you measure that?* Words like "chakra" or "didgeridoo" were part of casual conversation in therapy circles. I felt a bit on the outside—and not sure I wanted to come in. I didn't want to get lost on some esoteric path of soul retrieval or Shakti Goddess moon dances. But I was curious, and I needed some new tools to help the women on my couch.

I'd begun practicing Buddhism, a new job introduced me to Taoism, and a colleague taught me about Tantra. My love of literature introduced me to the secret world of Victorian sexuality. I read the *Kama Sutra*, met with experts on the feminine arts, interviewed an archeologist about an ancient culture of highly sexual women, investigated the lore of Caribbean women with a leading sexologist in the Dominican Republic, explored the sex appeal of Marilyn Monroe from her psychologist's point of view, and got inspired by the sensuality of poets and erotica.

Combining the wisdom of ancient cultures with the best of psychology, I began to form an approach uniquely my own. In *The Women on My Couch*, I wanted to honor women's sexuality by discussing it critically, exploring its nuances, and unraveling popular assumptions. No false promises of a mind-blowing sex life. No one particular sex practice as a panacea. Lust is a hothouse flower and requires careful attention. Not all women want the soft and fuzzies of intimacy, communication, and tenderness. When a frustrated client told me that she "wants to be ravaged," she was onto something. Unlikely qualities such as aggression, audacity, creativity, and leadership are essential for passion—as the client in my first chapter will discover.

My sojourn began with no friends, no job, and no plan. I showed up with few possessions. Only some clothing, most of which was too black and too formal for my new location. The journey had been a path well-worn: New York to California.

I'd arranged for a guy from a car dealership to pick me up at the airport. Sweaty and unhinged from an overnight flight, I sat in the back seat as a young man in a crisp uniform drove me to the dealership so

The Women on My Couch

I could purchase a car. The ride was battering bright, the sun's rays assaulting my sleepy eyes, accustomed to the shadows of Manhattan. I hadn't driven in six years. And I didn't give a rip about cars. I didn't want to be walked around the lot. Arriving to my new life felt too urgent to deal with superfluous details like stick shifts and power windows, so I simply said, "Give me the cheapest car you got."

"Well, don't you want to choose a color?" he asked.

"Pick one for me." I smiled.

I signed some paperwork, and thirty minutes later, I rolled out with a white Toyota Corolla.

I love start-overs. To honor the impulse to destroy your life. To walk away from your job, your lover, your friends, your possessions. I love the idea of self-reinvention; the possibility that exists in that space where no decision has yet been made. A new beginning is a chance to shed weight; the dull dissatisfactions and angst of unsolvable problems are stripped away, and a new uncertainty emerges—one filled with the best and worst the imagination has to offer. Sometimes a crisis gives you just that opportunity.

I'd never thought of moving to California. Well, I had fantasies of doing so, but my plan was to move to Florida to live with my boyfriend, Rami, after a six-year long-distance relationship. On the eve of my planned move, he balked and we broke up. My possessions were packed, my apartment lease terminated, and I'd said good-bye to the clients in my therapy practice. Suddenly, I had nowhere to go., but to be honest, I thrive in emergency situations, and a sort of crisis high buoyed me through the events to come.

I knew I was done with New York, my tiny apartment, and the lifestyle shared with my European friends with our constant smoking and red wine drinking. I wanted something more out of life than trendy bars and restaurants. I remember sitting in a bar, said red wine and cigarette in hand, explaining to my girlfriends that I wanted to be close to "Nature"—which was amusing to them. They were the kind of urban creatures who had no awareness that, standing beneath a redwood tree, one could look up and be moved to tears, propelled to wonder if ancient trees had souls or what the poet John Muir meant when he called Yosemite's Half Dome a sanctuary. I wanted to expand my horizon past the towers of metal and steel that had once evoked in me a similar awe. New York was starting to feel small.

I'd longed for an open vista, both literally and figuratively; to grow spiritually and intellectually and, of course, to find adventure. Pulling my new car onto the busy freeway, I had in hand three phone numbers of people who were renting out rooms. The first was an old Craftsman-style beach house full of surfer dudes, replete with beer cans and bongs and a big mess. They were friendly enough—but mentioned they could use a "female in the house." I tried not to laugh. I was probably messier than they were. The next house I went to visit, I simply couldn't find. My excitement and hope, the high of managing a crisis, were waning. Then, I pulled my car up to a large, pink, Spanish-style stucco home on a hillside across from a beach—a state park beach, no less. Nature!

I rang the doorbell, and a muscle-bound man, classically handsome with a California-carefree air, answered the door. He gave me a tour of the house and the outdoor seating areas framed by lush plants and flowers, each nook inviting me to read a book with a cup of tea, and a terraced garden dangling fresh vegetables. I said yes on the spot. For the first time in six years, I would live in a real house, like a real adult, with a living room that didn't double as kitchen or a bedroom.

As reality sank in a few weeks later, I began to feel the boundless, weightless effect of no routine, no immediate purpose. Heartbreak setting in, I began to run barefoot on the beach every morning. I was so awestruck by the rugged, dangerous beauty of the towering cliffs and violent, angry sea that swathed me in fresh foamy air that it was actually difficult to feel anything else. And it didn't hurt that as I woke up each morning I saw the glory of my handsome landlord—I mean, firemen-calendar kind of handsome—outside pulling weeds shirtless, bounding into the house with a handful of tomatoes for me. I somehow knew everything would be alright. He wouldn't become a love interest; in fact, he was nursing his own post-break-up wound. But he was, for me, a symbol that other men existed—something I'd been blind to for years.

The Women on My Couch

Every once in a while, my friends from New York would call and ask, "How's nature?" and start giggling. "Fucking awesome," I'd reply. I told them about the cliffs and the gleam of the sun on the blue sea at 8 a.m., about the smell of sage and the springtime coastal flowers—and my new life—beginning to bloom. At once excited and lovelorn, I began to receive my first clients.

The case studies in this book are inspired by real clients, but the true identities and backstories of the women have been fictionalized to protect their confidentiality. Stories were chosen based on their commonality rather than abnormality so that readers can relate and possibly find inspiration for their shared struggles. Also, the demographics of the clients are an actual representation of my clientele. As a result, women of all ages, ethnicities and gender identities are not equally represented.

Carla (Part 1)

Lying in bed, eyes heavy from the day, belly sated from dinner, she feels his hand reach over and cup her breast. That's when it sets in: rigor mortis. One simple change in sensation—his hand, gently treading upon her placid rest—and her body turns to stone. Now, she feels his breath near her face; he is leaning in to kiss her. A flash of irritation at this rude, interloping energy suddenly courses through her limbs as she realizes: *He wants to have sex.*

Carla doesn't want to resist. Yet she can't control this involuntary bracing. He's her boyfriend, the man she has spent a perfectly pleasant evening with, enjoying a dinner they cooked together, followed by snuggling and HBO. Now, as he starts to climb on top of her, she feels like she's suffocating under the weight—the heaviness of expectation, both his and hers. *Am I going to say no? Again? God, does his desire ever end?* She wants to sleep, but there are his feelings…*ugh. He will feel hurt, rejected.* She kisses him back, in that perfunctory way one does before leaving the house in the morning, and then rolls over.

By the time Carla made it to my office, the old "Not tonight, honey" line had been used one too many times, and the relationship had halted precariously on a single question: Can a sex drive be recovered?

Sitting on my couch, she looked at me expectantly, waiting for my answer. I felt a gust of anxiety, as I often do during these moments of urgent pause, when it's time for the expert to weigh in, my knowledge assumed to bear relief. But I didn't know if I could resuscitate her lust. Finding an answer, finding desire, would take time. My job is part archeologist and part experimental chef. I gazed back at her and then over at her boyfriend, who'd been silent.

Carla was Southern—and charming in the way only a Southern woman can be; the soft, halting tempo of her voice altered my perception of time, as if I was being lulled by a nymph. Her decorum and style must have taken great effort. I wished I had the patience for such grace.

Her Italian boyfriend, Sergio, sat next to her, his clothes pressed and shoes polished—not because his profession demanded it, but out of dignity. He was an anachronism, from a period when a man's charm derived from a combination of manners, masculinity, and vanity. I thought, *at face value, he's hot*. He looked like he could walk onto the set of *Mad Men*.

Carla faced a choice: have sex or lose the relationship. She'd run out of smooth excuses. There was no more avoiding his nightly proposal.

If the rest of us were like sloppy cursive, these two were like calligraphy. From outer appearances, they looked like they *should* want each other. Yet, attraction can be capricious, rude even. However, I believe the body is sentient—not just a dumb sack of meat designed to tote around our brilliant minds, but a real source of intelligence. I was curious about Carla's unwanted reaction. What was it communicating?

"If you could give a voice to that tension in your body when he makes a move, what would it say?" I asked her.

She paused.

"Get the fuck off me!"

Well, apparently her body had a bit of a different voice than the delicately cultivated one I'd been appreciating. She put her hand over her mouth.

"Don't shut yourself up. Be mean for a minute," I instructed. She removed her hand.

"It feels like a chore, but worse…I'd rather do chores. Fold laundry, do dishes, anything else. I do not want to have sex at all."

I won't accept clients that don't want a sex drive. I'm not in the business of telling women what they should be feeling, but Carla assured me that she wanted to want him, and that aside from her libido, she was happy in the relationship. This wasn't going to be an easy case, but I decided to give it a try.

Sexperts tell women like Carla that they should have sex even if they don't want to. This advice comes from the current therapy model on women's desire, which is the opposite of how most people assume sex works. The theory is that arousal, meaning lubrication, happens first, before desire. Or, let him touch you and hope it puts you in the mood. Not very exciting, I know, even though I've advised it. But if she doesn't want to "just do it," sexologists like to remind women that "withholding" is controlling and selfish; that never wanting sex is not an option in a relationship. There is truth in their advice, but tell "Miss Get the Fuck Off Me" to go through the motions? I couldn't think of a more absurd response to Carla's dilemma. I could have told her to "act as if," but to be honest, Carla already looked like she acted *as if* in many ways. Maybe this sleepy protest was one of her most authentic expressions.

Sergio feared that Carla was falling out of love with him, so he began to withdraw affection, hoping she'd figure out that he was unhappy with something. This ignoring behavior was, of course, a further turnoff. And did she figure it out? No. From her point of view, she now had a boyfriend who paid less attention to her yet still groped hungrily at her body every evening. I let him know that his strategy would lead to a sure breakup, and he agreed to give her affection—though he would only give without receiving for so long.

I continued my assessment by exploring her relationship to her sexuality.

"When *are* you in the mood?" I asked her.

"Honestly?" She raised her eyebrows. "Never."

"Do you masturbate?"

"Rarely."

"Think about sex with other men?"

"No."

"Not even Ryan Gosling?"

The Women on My Couch

"No."

"Ever in your whole life?"

I was prepared for another no. She wouldn't be the first to tell me that she had never been interested in sex.

"Four years ago, in the beginning of our relationship, we had sex all the time. Now, it's not on my mind. It doesn't bother me, though."

"What was your best sex like with Sergio?"

"I would tremble in his arms. When we kissed, I would inhale him."

"Did you have orgasms?"

"No. I didn't care. When he stopped intercourse to go down on me, it seemed like an interruption from the connection."

I understood the power of that experience, when an orgasm seems trifling in comparison to the passion, that sublime state where the body effortlessly welcomes, beckons even, inviting his essence to become part of her. It's an ecstasy of the soul that renders the motions of sex an inferior focus of attention.

Carla continued: "If I let him massage my clitoris, I'll be ready for sex, but I don't have enough interest to even allow it."

Carla knew the difference between arousal and desire. Arousal was a body experience; a brief, urgent tension that wanted release. Desire was a soul experience; one she wanted to savor and expand. Arousal could get her through the act, but it wasn't going to make her daydream about Sergio the next day.

Carla depended on romance to get turned on. This was a red flag. She lacked a connection to her own carnality. There was no animalistic impulse for fucking or playful impulse for titillation or creative impulse for eroticism—at least none that she was aware of—but I believed this could change. Romance is a narrow motive for sex, limiting the range of experience to one fickle feeling. It's not sustainable.

I wanted to see what would happen if I took Sergio out of the equation and guided her toward exploring her own instinct. I asked Carla to spend some time alone, read erotica, and just see if anything gave her a spark of desire.

Carla's experience of sex was a real departure from the soul rapture she'd just described. How was it that Sergio was all hot and bothered and she was…just *bothered*? These were such different trajectories for two people who had begun in the same place. Why this happens is a question that has troubled many great minds and marriages—and me; my practice was full of similar stories, and despite my expertise, I often felt as if I were sinking in quicksand.

The Internet is full of articles reporting on the research of evolutionary psychologists. Their perspective fits sexual behaviors into an evolutionary narrative, and they purport to have an answer for us. Yes, the long-awaited, categorical answer to a long-standing, complicated problem, drumroll……: *Women want sex less than men do.* It's a product of biology. Men are made to spread their seed, and women are discriminating and monogamy-loving. I'm shocked at how many therapists believe this explanation. Yes, desire dies for women. Often. Yet, there's one uncomfortable truth: their desire typically dies only for their husband or boyfriend. Women still get hot and bothered—for other men—a fact not included in these simple, sound-bite-ready studies.

I once attended a lecture at an esteemed psychological center in Los Angeles on this trendy approach to sex therapy. There, a room full of therapists, predominately women, were told by the professor, a middle-aged man, how important our youthful appearance and waist sizes were, and that if we don't measure up, not to worry, because men also value kindness. How gracious he was, to offer that condolence. At least there is always kindness.…

This professor also asserted that women are comfortable having sex with one partner for the rest of their lives, whereas men are freaked out by the idea. He even had slides with these dictates written out. Perhaps he could see many of the women in the audience shaking their heads and shifting in their seats, because he acknowledged aloud that this information would be uncomfortable to hear. But then he showed us another slide with just one phrase on it, as if to highlight its importance. The slide read, "Don't try to fight biology." It was as if he was saying, *you may not like it—but it's the truth.*

To see these ideas in concrete form, preached by a vaunted professor in a respected setting, had me fuming. I was about to stand up in confrontation, but one plucky elderly woman raised her hand and said, "This just doesn't seem modern; it's not what my clients are talking about."

She was right. My practice was full of women freaked out about monogamy, and men struggling with low libidos. I left wondering how this information was supposed to help my patients. Should I advise all the straight-waisted, small-lipped women with asymmetrical faces to learn how to specialize in kindness to make up for their unfortunate genetic situation? Should I tell the women who enjoy their marriages but have a low libido to just give up on trying to spice things up? The idea that a predetermined biology dictates sexual behavior doesn't leave room for change.

The notion that women are biologically less sexual than men was offensive to me. As if women were somehow deficient in the very force that propels all life, mere props for the fulfillment of men's urges. I thought, *Is that supposed to turn me on?* Clients don't want to hear that the stats are against them either. They want a solution. And I was determined to find one.

Sergio thought that because he wanted sex, Carla was the problem. It didn't occur to him that maybe he played a role in her not wanting sex. That perhaps he wasn't very seductive himself, that his initiation was lazy and boring and that he accepted her uninspired legs spreading and eyes closing for a real sexual experience—leaving her to further wonder about his intentions: *Does he not want that passion of our early years? Is this what he prefers? Just to get off and go to sleep?* Sergio decided that Carla wasn't normal and sent her to me. He only wanted to come in periodically for a progress report. She agreed to this without reservation.

I didn't mind starting therapy this way. It may not have been fair, but the pressure was on her, and that wasn't necessarily a bad thing. If I could effect change in her, he was bound to have a reaction. I was sure I'd be seeing him again.

I suspected that beneath the façade of this perfect-looking couple, there would be some intriguing hidden reasons why her flesh was turning into pavement. Libido is a barometer. It tells you, in painfully accurate measure, that something is wrong, regardless of whether you want to see it.

Carla arrived for our next appointment alone. She arranged my pillows to her liking, leaned back into the couch, and smiled, signaling she was ready to begin. I sat, silent for a moment, waiting for her to take the lead, assuming one's goals are self-determined. Instead of speaking, she gazed at me expectantly. This little act of deference could be interpreted as emblematic of how she approaches sex, men, or anything. I wondered if I should address it, but decided not to.

"Did you do the homework assignment?" I asked.

"I'm so sorry—I forgot. What was it?" she said in a way that sounded like *I'm sorry, who are you again?* She removed the sunglasses from the top of her head and placed them in her Gucci bag, withdrawing eye contact.

"I had asked you to read some erotica, to see if you had any reaction to it," I said, holding my gaze.

"Aren't those books kind of corny?" she said imperiously.

"You seemed so motivated about coming to therapy, and then you forget to do the first homework assignment—something doesn't measure up."

"I'm sorry, I meant to do it. I just had a busy week."

I leaned forward.

"Carla, why are you here?"

"Because it's the one issue that's preventing him from proposing."

"So, what happens after you achieve that goal? You'll still have this guy wanting to have sex with you every night for the rest of your life."

"Oh my God." She rolled her eyes.

"Maybe you didn't do the homework because you're not doing it for you. Do you care if you want sex or not?"

"Not really."

"Good to know. We need to start with the truth. How often do you think it's valuable to have sex for the purpose of keeping him?"

"Maybe once a week."

"OK, let's start there. Would you rather enjoy that once a week, or would you rather feel like you are toiling in a labor camp?"

"I understand, but homework assignments feel like work. Sex should be spontaneous."

"If you find sex to be a chore, nothing is going to be spontaneous except sleep. You claim to still love him, yet you are fine thinking that this intimate act is a boring chore. Do you want to feel that way about physically connecting to the man you want to spend your life with?"

Carla was so close to getting what she wanted—a wedding—that she had lost concern for the quality of their relationship. Her mind was all dusty roses in mason jars, and crab in cream sauce served over grits, and mermaid dress versus ball gown. But a woman's sex drive is only sustainable when she can tap into her own intrinsic motivation, not when she's doing it as a means to an end.

It didn't surprise me that Carla ditched the homework. Until this moment, she'd done a lot of complaining or head-nodding in agreement. I had edged myself up next to her limits, and now I could see that she was a real person. Her petulant resistance was a form of honesty. Carla fought an internal battle with being polite yet wishing she were uninhibited. She wasn't the type of person who commanded a room with charisma, but you'd know she was there; she might not tell the waiter he forgot to put the dressing on the side, but she was in a mid-level managerial position at work, so she was at least intermittently capable of knowing what she wanted and telling that to the world. But when it came to sex, Carla disappeared. She followed Sergio's lead, rarely initiated, spoke a word, or shared a fantasy. When she had sex, she was either full of love or full of resentment—and Sergio never knew the difference.

The women in my practice are a mix of ages and religious backgrounds, yet many of them share in Carla's bored, placating style. Most, in fact, aren't religious and are ideologically tolerant of sexual diversity, and some have had wild sexual adventures in their past—yet are still indifferent and passive with their boyfriends. Did liberation bring us more orgasms but no desire? Lusty women populate movies, porn, and feminist erotica; women initiate sex, seduce, enjoy orgasms, and take many lovers. Yet there is a discrepancy between media and real life. Were the evolutionary theorists correct? Maybe female desire is an ideal of equality between the sexes that isn't real in nature. Was I forcing the idea?

Sex therapy is successful in treating most bedroom complaints, but when it comes to sex drive—there is no effective treatment. One study even found that improving emotional connection and communication had the opposite result: people were even less attracted to each other. I was beginning to question my choice of specialty. Didn't I want to treat something for which I could offer reliable relief? Like a panic disorder or OCD? Despite the plethora of spice-it-up books promising to fill women with a new spark, those of us in practice know the truth: the advice rarely works. Some days I thought the monogamy cynics, polyamorists, swingers, and serial monogamists had the right answer—adapting to a reality the rest of us wanted to deny. Despite the lack of personal gratification, I couldn't avoid the question of desire and what makes this elusive force work—the force that drives us to write poetry, risk our lives for an affair, or succumb to bleakness when the thrill is gone. This question of desire was really my search for possibility, an answer to provide when confronted with those expectant eyes. And my need for hope had set me upon an unexpected adventure.

I realized that I needed to change my path when I was trained to use the standard sex therapy homework assignments developed by the famed 1960s research team Masters and Johnson. Their techniques, which focused on touch and sensation, were effective in fixing problems with orgasms and organs, but they lacked soul. Couples in my office protested these assignments because they didn't give them what they really wanted: the throbbing of want, the sweet ache of yearning, transcendence. My feelings crystalized when I interviewed for a position at a sex research lab. Its stark white walls and big machines with electrodes that hooked up to people's genitals while they watched porn, and the lab technicians who measured their lubrication or tumescence, told me about the state of psychology and sex. The place felt like you were going for a gynecological exam on the Starship *Enterprise*. I don't know what I should have expected. Red velvet curtains, low-slung couches, Al Green in the background? But I looked around and thought: *Psychology isn't sexy. If I'm not turned on, I'm doing it wrong.* I decided to search elsewhere for understanding. I was tired of parsing out the problem. I wanted inspiration. I wanted to know the full potential of a woman's desire. I wanted examples of women who radiated sensuality. I needed my own modern-day Aphrodite, and that became my quest—to find her.

If I could find some Aphrodite's, then I could use inspiration as a tool in therapy. A great deal of learning takes place through the process of internalizing what we see in our environment. Our modern world is full of sexualized images, but most are idealized images of sex appeal, not the authentic yearnings of a woman's soul—or loins. We're surrounded by scripts of what men want. While Sergio's needs are important, Carla has to discover her own unique lust. Finding desire is finding voice; a form of personal development and a form of power. In fact, a woman fully embodied in her desire has been proven so powerful that throughout history, there have been efforts to shut down desire by the institutions (religions, governments) of many countries. Desire is political. So, in the therapy room with a woman like Carla, whose motivation remains low despite the high stakes in her relationship, I find myself in the position of having to convince her why it's important, why desire isn't for him, why it's not frivolous titillation. Desire matters. And it's worth fighting for.

I set out to explore as far and wide as I could: from the ancient arts of seduction found in the *Kama Sutra* to the Taoist texts of loving, to modern-day erotica writers and gurus of the female orgasm. I sat down with a stack of history books, traveled, and conducted interviews.

I learned that other places and times had solutions to our modern sexual dilemmas, everything from libido to sexual fetishes. Psychology must be understood in the context of history and culture if we want to evolve. Yes, we have a long record of repression. We've heard it all before; but if we take that historical fact, then play the tape backward, what do we see?

Here lies the untold story: women with a higher libido than men. Women who mastered the arts of seduction. Women who knew how to love better.

This life-changing wisdom that I encountered I would now apply to Carla's situation.

Carla (Part 2)

Good sex begins with the imagination. I keep a collection of erotic stories in my office and have clients do readings. They picture themselves in the fantasies, explore their reactions, and find inspiration. When Carla returned for the next session, she flounced through the door and pulled a book from her purse, pride flashing in her hazel eyes. She'd bought her own erotica book.

I raised an eyebrow.

"I got turned on," she said, and tittered. "I liked one about a business owner who commanded an employee to please him. He was very authoritative."

She flashed me a little side smile. I was relieved to hear that she liked something, anything.

"What if Sergio talked to you like that?"

"I don't know if he could. He's very tender, sweet."

"So you stay silent?"

"Yes. I don't want him to feel bad."

"But the consequence is that nobody is present. If you were talking, at least you'd both be there in the interaction."

"Yes, but to break the silence would seem so strange. What would he think if I asked for something different? Or what if he can't pull it off, and it doesn't turn us on? Then we'll be faced with the realization that nothing is going to help us, that we can't find any attraction."

I empathized with the gravity of this fear. It can be paralyzing. But I knew the choice made in this very moment would impact the course of her relationship, and her life.

"I don't know what I want. As I was reading the erotica stories, I kept thinking, *I can't be that—it's not me*. I think I'd feel silly."

"So, eroticism is silly."

"I don't want to be on stage."

"OK, so just hide."

She shrugged.

"You can't go fetal anymore. You have to show up."

She collapsed her shoulders and lowered her head, sinking away from me. Away from herself. I knew she wasn't ready to "show up," but I needed her to see the goal.

Sadly, this is where therapy for low libido typically fails; a refusal to be seen. Exciting sex requires putting yourself out there. Sexually, she was disembodied, embarrassed, and afraid to step into the power of her own eroticism. I asked if she could imagine masturbating in front of him—as a symbol of her ability to present her sexuality to him. She said that idea mortified her.

Change requires a leap. Carla was standing at the deep end and I was asking her to jump in. I was really rooting for her. I was also aware of Sergio's feelings. His sense of urgency was now directed at me. He'd send me emails, telling on her for not reading the erotica books or for not wearing sexy clothes to bed (not a homework assignment—but an act that held significance for him). His rejection anxiety was becoming intolerable, and so to de-escalate the situation, I validated his position. I acknowledged the difficulty of sex being the one thing you can't get outside of a marriage—unless one opts for infidelity, an open relationship, or a hall pass (a one-time, preapproved tryst with another). If sex isn't happening and your partner isn't content, the issue can't be ignored. It's normal for a couple to have a difference in libido, just as it's normal for people to have different levels of desire for anything from having a child to having a vacation. What's important is how couples deal with that difference.

I asked Sergio to stop initiating sex for one month so Carla could have some space to connect to her own sensuality. I told him that it helps if he's not "waiting" like a panting retriever. I couldn't tell if she had intimacy issues or if he was needy. He agreed to give her space and said that if the matter of sex could be solved, he was prepared to propose marriage.

I now had one month, a short time, so I advised that Carla begin a daily practice. I sent her home with a prescription to spend time nude with a mirror, gazing, masturbating, and affirming—all to build a foundation of comfort with her own body. Yet, one can't just become a fully actualized sex whiz by decision alone—especially if her baseline is "get the fuck off me."

Carla needed a new vision for herself. I wanted to provide inspiration; an Aphrodite figure that could stand as a symbol for what she was capable of becoming. Again, I would use an erotica book, the diary of Cora Pearl.

In 1864 Paris, the era's most flamboyant courtesan, Cora Pearl, made an unforgettable entrance—an entrance talked about all over town. Men of title filled the dining room, and waited. Seated around a dining table at the famed salon she hosted, a nobleman, a military leader, and even a prince conversed as they awaited the final course. From the kitchen, a large, covered silver tray was carried out by two footmen and placed at the center of the table. "When the lid was lifted," the diary recalls, "I was rewarded by finding myself the center of a ring of round eyes and half open mouths."

Reclining on her side, head in hand, Cora Pearl lay nude, her body covered in cream sauce. Her breasts were dusted in powdered sugar and adorned with tiny rosette wreaths. A single grape bedecked her navel.

Once the shock wore off, one gentleman casually removed the grape and "slipped it slowly between his lips." Then, the men feasted upon her body.

I was intrigued by the notorious antics of the 19th century French courtesans, but I wasn't sure if there was a lesson about libido for the modern woman. What could a courtesan know about the tedious side of monogamy?

Courtesans inhabited mansions, gilded and marbled. They bathed in champagne and wore designer gowns daily. The modern woman doesn't have a team of servants or a personal chef. We don't have a handmaiden to follow us around holding a pillow of jewels so we can change out a ruby for a diamond in the middle of a cocktail party. Nor can we sit around all day and read the *Economist*, practice the piano, write some poetry, then put on a corset and host a dinner. It takes time and money to make this scene happen.

However, once I learned more about the historical context the courtesans inhabited, I realized that I'd come across some important insights about lust. To ascend to the rank of a courtesan was rare. The affections of the capricious men of the aristocracy drew fierce competition, leading courtesans to perfect the art of inciting desire. Cora Pearl devised her grand entrance after a rival dominated Paris gossip when she "invited a coterie of her most influential admirers to her apartment, and received them sitting in a bath of milk. Rising from this bath in a manner most calculated to expose her charms, she had summoned a pair of *filles de ferme* who had dried her with the most lascivious gestures and displays, whereupon she had withdrawn, leaving her audience in a fever of unassuaged lust."

Cora Pearl's career was rife with outrageous acts of eroticism. Shortly after meeting some duke, she told him of her wish to have more horses. As a gesture of admiration, he sent an Arab horse. When he showed up unexpectedly and she wasn't prepared to receive him, she quickly stripped off all of her clothes and rode out on the new horse to demonstrate her prowess as a master horsewoman. She rode up close to him, and as he attempted to help her dismount, she said, "No, sir, just as a horse needs care after exercise, so I need to bathe and rest. But be assured that your gift will be acknowledged by my lasting admiration." She then rode off back to her stable, leaving him there to drool.

To be a good lover requires risk and courage. The lesson from Cora Pearl is not that we should arrive to our next dinner party on a platter. These tales are a metaphor about the audacity to be seen. Too outlandish to be taken literally, they instead bring up questions that are useful

for the contemporary women. In what ways are we comfortable being seen? Can we allow others to see our emotions? Our bodies? Our
erotic side? What do we cover up and why?

Boredom is monogamy's greatest threat. I knew Carla wasn't going
to be "outrageous" anytime soon, nor was that my goal for her. But I
wanted her to read these stories and imagine herself as bold. Courtesans
created a sublime space for eroticism with an extravagance that wasn't
just about wealth; it was the ceremony that made the display of their
sexuality a special event. Cora was famous for her attention to detail;
the food, the fabric, the flowers, the scents and lingerie were all calculated to create a superlative experience. I thought about Carla and
Sergio. This wasn't happening between dinner and HBO. For Sergio
and Carla, there was no art, seduction, or ambience. Most importantly,
there was no audacity—and love wasn't enough.

My new office was located in a neighborhood next to Hollywood. A
hilly community populated by writers, artists, and musicians living in
old Spanish Mediterranean homes painted pink, orange, and turquoise.
Lemon trees, cacti, pomegranates, palms, and colorful blooms dangled
and delighted at every turn of the winding steep hills and their secret
stairways. There were hipsters of varying degrees of solvency—depending on how high up the hill they lived—mixed with gangsters
occasionally shooting each other in the midst of the gritty paradise.
Taking walks in between clients, I would notice how the gangsters and
hipsters passed each other on the street, neither seemingly interested in
the other, both lost in their own ambitions. I disliked the neighborhood
at first. I was too distracted by the garishness of junky strip malls, auto-
repair shops, and storefront Dentista's to appreciate the trendy coffee
shops set in between. My office had a view of the Hollywood sign,
perched in the hills of Griffith Park, tempting inhabitants to dream
another day. Most of my view, however, was blocked by a Del Taco sign.
A man was shot and killed in front of that Del Taco just the day before.
I struggled to accept the constant duality of L.A.—the ugliness and
beauty, the hopes and injustices, always visible.

Carla showed up for her next appointment feeling accomplished. She'd initiated sex with a small gesture that was a big step for her. She had surprised Sergio by waking him up in the morning with a blow job. This, of course, put him in a pleasant mood. She noticed that for the rest of the day he was more attentive.

"An astute connection." I laughed.

She laughed, then said, "I hate that he requires that to be in a good mood."

"Did you like it?"

"It's uncomfortable—I get tired."

"So you just plowed through it to make him happy?"

I had hoped she would get aroused, but she was satisfied that he was happy.

"I had this moment during, when I was thinking…*What am I doing here? This is so weird. I'm sticking his body part into my head repetitively*."

"You had a meta-moment. It's fine. Use it as a moment of choice. See if you can think about what's sexy about it."

"I don't know—I guess I've always looked at it as degrading. Something that guys want but the woman doesn't really."

"All that matters in the moment is your gaze. What you choose to think. What if we could change what that act means to you? Even if that negative way of looking at blow jobs is all around us?"

What made Cora Pearl so appealing? She was widely described as having perfect, ample breasts and plain face which she overpainted in compensation. She looks beautiful to me in the few photographs I've seen. However, what stood out in my research was her attitude. She's described as witty and full of gaiety and kindness. The erotica text describes her approach to sex.

"He had given me the most soothing and beguiling attention, he turned to my sex and with great skill manipulated it to the point of utmost pleasure. As he was doing this, delighted by the muscular thigh only a little away from my lips, I could not resist plunging my hand beneath his loincloth…."

The Women on My Couch

Regardless of what her patrons looked like—and some were described as hairy, fat, stinky men—her attitude was replete with joy, acceptance, and kindness. She beheld the male body with reverence and appreciation as if fulfilling its pleasures were her spirituality. She seemed to do this without any sense of servility. She seemed as if she would meet an erection with alacrity.

Women are used to being admired for their beauty—and we forget the importance of seeing the beauty in *his* body, in *his* desires. And the cost is a lowered libido. The first question in my mind when a woman doesn't want to have sex with her man is: *Has she turned herself off with a negative view of him, or of men in general?*

When Cora met a bad lover, rather than holding him in contempt, she relished in teaching him how to touch a woman. I noticed in my practice that women tended to be more intolerant when men weren't great lovers. With disdain, they'd complain that men are awkward, clumsy, too rough or too gentle, can't finish or can't keep it up. I'm sure it's all true. Yet, I rarely hear men speak this way about their lovers. If he doesn't know where and how to touch her, it's her fault—and so are the negative judgments.

"Nature has made me the happiest of receivers of sensual pleasure; and fortunately too, the mode of life I have enjoyed has enabled me to teach the gentlemen who have come to me much about the art of love."

Surely, this must have been more exciting for the patron—to be with a woman who was authentically into it. Perhaps her lure was that her desire wasn't counterfeit. I think Cora understood that sex isn't about giving something away. A blow job is neither charity nor a chore. She seemed very present and embodied, herself receiving something from the interaction, something more than money or love: a mutual sortie in carnal decadence.

Carla needed to see the magnificence in Sergio's body. To see his face, his chest, his penis as beauty. To gaze upon his body, his sexual desire with the same awe typically reserved for the sky or the sea or mountains. Or at least remember to notice how hot the guy looks in a suit. Attitude change on this foundational level, the base from which one perceives the ideas of sex, love or men, takes more time than most of my clients expect. Approaching attitude change as if it's a singular decision is like trying to remove a permanent tattoo with soap and water. New learning is possible, but it's more like a full-on self-propaganda campaign, brainwashing oneself into the new way of thinking. But audacity is not a mental exercise. It takes action. *If audacity is for the desperate,* I thought, *Carla is ripe for it.*

Instead of just talking about her apathy, I had Carla try out new ways of being. I had her write a fantasy and read it out loud in my office, calming herself with her breath each time she felt anxious, and speaking more slowly when she disconnected. I had her read aloud a list of sexual words—*lick, suck, fuck*—over and over until she was desensitized to them. I had her do that while looking in the mirror. I had her walk slowly around my office, paying attention to her body, learning to live in it. I asked her to appreciate her various body parts, then to walk as if she were feeling that appreciation. I used visualizations. I had her read various poems, from the spiritual to the natural to the kinky—and give me a reaction. It turned out that she hated the flowery Chinese poems but loved the ravenous Pablo Neruda. She hated the ideas of Tantra and felt indifferent toward the leading, lustful female protagonists, but she found her niche in stories with a light BDSM theme, in particular the ones with leading men—or multiple men. She was beginning to develop her own set of preferences.

In a relationship, it's easy to forget yourself. You spend so much time bending, flowing, weaving into your partner's rhythms and desires, erasing the parts of you that don't blend, that you lose a sense of grounding. This happens sexually too; you have your routines, or an agreed-upon script—or one that was his all along—and you follow out of expediency.

The day of our next couple's appointment was a heatstroke-hot kind of day. With the lush vegetation of my neighborhood, it's easy to forget that Southern California is a desert. Most apartment buildings are old and don't have air conditioning. So you open your windows, put your hair in a bun, wear a tank with no bra, and sweat for five months. This could be sexy, but today, the ruthless sunshine made me irritable and putting a light blouse on for work felt like wool. I went to my office. I was a few minutes late. Carla came in; Sergio came with her, for his progress report. Both were smiling. They looked cool. I assumed they lived up the hill—where homes have air conditioning.

Carla and Sergio shared with me that on the way home from a bar one night, they stopped by a sex toy store on Hollywood Boulevard. She loaded up on toys and picked out a black spandex mini-dress. At home, Carla put the dress on while Sergio lit candles in the living room and played a White Stripes CD. He took a seat on the couch, with a glass of Scotch in hand. Carla emerged, and walked toward him slowly, pausing to pose and dance in a way she remembered from a burlesque show; but she teetered in her heels and felt unsure of how to move her body, so she took a breath and sat down on the couch opposite him. Her voice shaking, she announced that she was a peep-show girl and that he had to maintain his distance. For the next thirty seconds, she would do anything he wanted. First he had to place the cash on the table. Sergio smiled, pulled out his wallet, and asked her to show off the back of her dress. Carla crawled on the couch like a cat, arching her back and swiveling her hips, showing off the sleek spandex that barely covered her backside.

"Time's up," said Carla. "Why don't you put some more money down, and tell me what you like."

He smiled and put more down. Carla sat forward on the couch, slowly inching her legs open, maintaining eye contact. She felt so exposed and anxious, but she could see that Sergio was into it. She began to touch herself and said, "I'd like to show you my body. Why don't you come a little closer?" He moved across the living room, over to her. "Kneel down," she said. "Lick." She allowed herself to surrender to receiving. And finally, she felt pleasure. She had a few moments of wondering if he was enjoying himself—which he was—and remembered her right to pleasure. "Get up," she said. "Now I want you inside me." He complied. He began to move feverishly, and she grew exhilarated, her body full of pleasure.

Then he began to slow down, to control himself, and she whispered, "I want you to spank me." But he didn't; he paused for an uncomfortable minute. Instead, he whispered in her ear, "I adore you."

"Pull my hair," she said, before noticing that he had lost his erection. He pulled out and lay next to her. She had just gotten into it, had felt that desire pulsing through. It had taken a while; she'd felt staged and sort of out-of-body, but then she had really let go and felt so alive. Her body wanted action—she wanted to buck and writhe into his masculinity. She wanted him to grab at her flesh. Instead, he was softly stroking her arm.

What had happened? Why did he freeze? The turning point was when she asked him to show some aggression.

Sergio explained, "I don't know why women want that *Fifty Shades* stuff. I didn't feel like hitting her. I was in a different place. More adoring, soft. I thought that's what women want."

"Women want to get fucked," said Carla.

"It's not who I am. I hate macho stereotypes," he said.

He had a point about women's expectations of masculinity. But I was curious about the sudden desire to cuddle. I recognized this as what Freud called "libidinal regression"—when sexual anxiety triggers a regression back to the safety of spooning and *I love you boo-boos*. I hypothesized that Carla coming out of her shell had unnerved him.

I've had a legion of men through my office telling me that they like the submissive role—and that the women in their lives don't want to play the dominant role for them. I've seen this gender role reversal lead to rage from both sides. Some blame feminists—that they've turned men into saps who can't get it up. But this phenomenon has been documented since long before women's equality. So what if a guy wants to play that role? We've been socialized into very strict roles, which we've had a couple hundred years to internalize into our psyches. Is his passivity pathological? It's hard to say. There is great pleasure in surrender; also great laziness. Passivity can be a comfort zone for those afraid to be an active participant in the experience.

Where does this story that men are more sexual and dominant than women come from? That we are passive and men aggressive, the ones who express desire overtly—while we only express it in a coy, seductive manner, if at all? Is this Mother Nature, as the evolutionary theorists propose? Guys like Sergio don't fit this story. Nor do the many women I come across who are sexually ravenous and bold.

I had once lost sexual interest in a long-term relationship and I realized that I shared with Carla many of the same expectations that men should take all the actions—until I began to read. Never before had a reading of historical facts been more emotionally gripping for me. What felt like a personal failure turned out to be a symptom of a history that I shared with millions of women. Just a brief peek into the history of Western sexuality places all of our current assumptions about what it means to be sexually powerful or passive under question.

Cora Pearl lived in a decisive time in the history of sexuality. Her story provides a powerful lesson about what happened to desire and a woman's potential. Like most young women of her time, she went to school in a Catholic convent. Her family had planned for her to work in millinery and hoped for the prospect of marriage. Because she was raised in a port town full of sailors and merchants, the sex trade flourished in the streets, dance halls, and brothels. Men and women were hustling sex out in the open, in broad daylight, so Cora rarely left the house alone. On one of the rare occasions when she walked outside unchaperoned, she was seduced by a stranger, then drugged and raped. She knew the next morning that she had just given up her prospects for marriage. A grim reality faced her: hard labor in a factory or prostitution.

Cora's decision wasn't radical at the time. To understand her choice and how it impacts the story of Carla and Sergio, I'll provide a truncated summary of how libido was hijacked. Prostitution flourished almost everywhere in Paris due to a massive influx of industrial workers into the city. Solicitation in the street—an act of survival—was largely viewed as licentious rather than what it really was: a wage issue. Nineteenth-century Paris was actually a grim place. The average woman worked: in factories and mills, and as maids and seamstresses. Wages were so low that many working women still lived in poverty, so turning to prostitution was common. And glamorous it was not. For many, it involved the risk of contracting a disease, begging, and enduring disrespect. Women could not own property, so at best, an unmarried working woman could try to find a man to pay her rent in exchange for some combination of sex and romance.

The aristocracy and middle classes of the time tried to socially differentiate themselves by establishing decorum that stressed moral values, order, and restraint of impulses. Every realm, from media to religion, broadcast these values, eventually inculcating the entire population with this point of view. Girls were largely educated by the Catholic Church and socialized to believe that expression of sexual desire was contemptible. They were taught to demonstrate innocence, for showing any knowledge of sex would be suspicious and impact marriageability. Therefore, acting unsexual was a determinant of her life's outcome. Virginity and fidelity were essential because they played a role in preserving the transfer of property among family dynasties. Acting sexually unenthusiastic was lauded, a source of pride and superiority.

Motherhood was romanticized, but marriages weren't about passion. I'm sure lots of married people loved each other, but being "in love" wasn't the standard for marriage. Further, a sexual relationship, beyond procreation, between husband and wife wasn't the norm. When I think about the love lives of young nineteenth-century French women, who weren't supposed to be out dating or hooking up and then ended up in these sexless marriages, I imagine I would have developed hysteria for sure. Even in marriage, women were supposed to maintain purity, not inciting desire in their husbands and not seeking out pleasure at all.

The poor (especially single women, who worked and sold their bodies) were pathologized as being chaotic, dangerous, and animalistic. Sex workers and ultimately, by extension, any woman expressing sexual assertiveness became associated with one of the most powerful inhibitors of behavior known to humans: shame. Consider that the biological function of shame is to shape social behavior with a feeling of aversion, which prevents us from doing things that would have us potentially rejected from the pack. Shame even encodes differently into memory, so that we can easily recall experiences of it in order to continue inhibiting that behavior in the future. So, this attachment of shame to sex for women was a mighty turn in human history. Collectively and individually, we must all overcome *learned shame.*

Desire is influenced by storytelling. What a woman feels is influenced by the social meaning of our cultural stories about sex and sex appeal. What is shamed and what is praised are the products of cultural attitudes. We must be aware of who controls the narrative about what a sexual woman looks like. The angelic versus the savage street woman is still woven into the American psyche. It's important to note that this narrative has a beginning, and it's not with Adam and Eve. When put into historical perspective, it's a new story. In fact, the idea that women have a lower sex drive than men; that we're supposed to be passive or coy or innocent or romantic, is only a few hundred years old.

Before the Victorian era, women across Europe and beyond were known as sexually voracious. This is the untold story—that before the altering of our gaze, limiting it to this one particular dichotomy, there existed a world where women lusted. A woman's pleasure was thought to be necessary for conception—and, therefore, important. Sex manuals emphasized clitoral orgasms long before Freud declared them "immature." A manual in the seventeenth century thought to be the authority on sex and birth, called *Aristotle's Masterpiece* (written by an anonymous author posing as Aristotle who was thought for a long time to be *the* expert on sex), declared that if a woman is deprived of sex, she becomes a "green and weasel coloured" old maid. A well-sexed *and* well-loved woman was necessary for procreation. Eventually, people discovered that a woman's pleasure wasn't actually necessary and soon, the woman's orgasm, and the necessity of love, fell out of favor, even came to be seen as sort of backward and ignorant. The longstanding *Masterpiece* became thought of as lewd.

Carla took Sergio to a neighborhood French café, brought Cora's diary, and read it to him in a low voice over a bottle of wine. She teased him in between passages and whispered about what she'd do to him later.

Carla (Part 2)

Sergio loved Cora Pearl and loved the new Carla even more. She was expanding her limits and now it was his turn to grow. I've noticed in my practice that sexual inhibition and anxiety are not unique to women. I explained this history to Sergio and Carla so they could understand that the roles they played were fabricated and were where they began. Men, too, have been held captive by this history, deprived of their own range of expression. Sergio wanted his chance to surrender without being judged. The norms of male dominance have been eroticized and held in the collective unconscious, thus creating ambivalence about venturing outside what feels "natural." They each had to take a risk at breaking from convention—just like Cora did.

Cora Pearl and the courtesans are historically important because in an environment of rigid propriety and duty, these ladies kept sensuality alive. Ms. Pearl was widely viewed in her time as reckless and extravagant, but as she made her ostentatious appearances on the promenades of Paris, she was defying the Church's strictures in a time when women couldn't vote or own property and weren't fully educated. It was a sexy act of civil disobedience. She stood for pleasure against all the forces that tried to shut it down, even when she was publicly shamed. So, when we are tempted to think that sensuality is a frivolous pursuit, historical hindsight reminds us that pleasure is an issue of economics, politics, and a civil society.

As for the fate of France's ladies of the street, the government vacillated between legalizing and criminalizing prostitution, and eventually women were rounded up and held in prison because a government official had a new idea. Put them all on a ship and send their decadence and immorality away from France forever, to a remote outpost: New Orleans.

Cora became broke and died of cancer in the south of France. She'd lost her place in society after the Franco-Prussian War upended the aristocracy that had supported her. When many of her benefactors had fled the country, she stayed during the siege of Paris and turned her opulent mansion into a hospital, hiring a medical staff to serve the wounded. The injured men, some dying, others who'd lost a limb, would reach up for the breasts of the nurses caring for them, about which Cora wrote: "I encouraged the girls to give of themselves freely…truly love is one of the most powerful human emotions."

Like Cora Pearl, women need to be accountable for pursuing their sexual development because men aren't going to hand it to us on a platter—although, like Sergio, many men are willing to provide support.

Anyone can ride the high of chemistry in the beginning of a relationship. Once that dies down, one's actual sexual capacity is exposed. Do we hide our fantasies, close our eyes and say nothing? Do we hide our lust out of embarrassment? Sexual actualization is connected to self-actualization. The Cora Pearl tale is a parable for a sexually mature woman; a woman who takes the leadership role in the bedroom, a woman who knows what she wants and feels entitled to direct the evening, and finally, a woman with the courage to stand tall in the vulnerability of being seen. Or to recline in dignity while covered in cream sauce and powdered sugar.

Carla and Sergio agreed to experiment with new roles. Carla admitted that she enjoyed becoming more assertive. It was a bumpy road, as her impulses chafed against his. They didn't recover the glory of their early passions, but their sex had life again, and in that sometimes troublesome weaving together of two desires, they found a new level of intimacy. As a result of being more sexual, Carla had found her loving and appreciative feelings toward Sergio again. There was no more rigor mortis.

Carla decided to end therapy when she got what she wanted.

She came for that final session elated, gliding into my office in a flowing orange dress.

"I've got to tell you something. We got engaged!" she announced, holding out her hand to show off her gleaming diamond set in a vintage platinum band.

"Mermaid or ball gown?" I asked.

"Mermaid."

Fair enough, I thought. This was a realistic outcome for therapy. Carla wasn't going to become the next Cora Pearl, but she'd made real progress. As for me, I thought I'd found a pretty awesome Aphrodite figure. Reading Cora's diary was inspiring and erotic, and the French history had mobilized me to rise out of a legacy of lethargy, to become more daring. But how would I teach this? There was no concrete skill set to learn here. For that, I would have to turn to the East: India and China.

*There are multiple versions of Cora Pearl's diary, as well as 19th century Parisian newspapers that describe her notorious antics. It's difficult to parse out what is rumor, truth or embellishment as courtesans thrived on the rumor mill of the society pages, using their outrageous acts to gain popularity. The version that I use with my clients is a work of erotic literature, an embellished version called **Grand Horizontal: Memoirs of Cora Pearl,** written by William Blatchford, a.k.a Derek Parker. I chose to focus on this book because the value of these tales is metaphorical rather than literal. For my purposes, they are meant to be read as parables for understanding The Erotic Woman as an archetype that anyone can access from within. For details and facts about the life of Cora Pearl, read **The Memoirs of Cora Pearl** by Cora Pearl or **The Pearl from Plymouth** by Wilfred Holden.*

Isabella

They met in narrow bar with a band too large and too loud for the space. A man pushed through the crowd. Isabella was in his way. He grabbed her by the hips. She turned, and then smiled when she saw a handsome face. He pushed her up against the wall and lifted her up. Then, slowly, he slid her down and whispered in her ear, "You," and walked away. Isabella lingered for a moment, and then joined her friends. When she could, she'd steal a glance around the room but didn't see him again.

After leaving the bar a few hours later, she rested against a mailbox to remove her heels and looked up. The handsome stranger was standing against the wall smoking a cigarette, his eyes, ink black and boldly rude.

"I need a man to carry me," said Isabella, standing barefoot on the concrete sidewalk.

He came over and hoisted her up on his back.

"Where to, my lady?"

"The deli. I want a sandwich."

She ordered a sandwich while sitting on his back and they walked back out to the street.

"Do you like being carried?"

"Yes."

"If you stay on my back, then you have no choice where I take you. Do you agree?"

"Yes."

They walked past the vagrants and tweekers and high-end galleries of downtown Los Angeles. It was summer, night, and the air felt like warm

34

butter on her skin. He decided to climb the fire escape of a nearby building. Without knowing names or dreams or fears, driven only by a primal certitude, they began clawing at each other's bodies on the roof-top. Now, a month later, they stayed in his bed on Sunday afternoons, failing to get up because nothing was more compelling than touching and talking about nothing.

At 42, Isabella was recently divorced and had been flirting her nights away at restaurants and lounges, waiting for texts, scanning Tinder, and fielding emails from men. She'd felt invisible to her husband for years. She could put on a tight dress, have her hair done, and he'd barely glance at her. It was such a terrible feeling, to know she had become the woman a man was tired of fucking. Isabella felt that she, her very essence, was an empty milk carton, crushed and tossed in the trash.

Now, lying in bed with her younger lover, a musician named Keis, her spirit was soaring. Between teasing about her cold feet and a triangle of freckles near her belly button, he whispered, "Tell me, Madame, that I'm your slave."

"You're my slave," Isabella repeated, her tone lacking authority.

"Madame, tell me what to do to you," he continued.

Slightly embarrassed that she sounded tremulous, she decided to go with it. She affected a serious face.

"Suck my nipple," she directed.

He did.

"Tell me that you'll punish me if I don't get it right."

Keis was teaching her some kind of script that he liked. Isabella wasn't in the mood for this game, but she wanted to please him. She liked that he was sharing his fantasy with her. There was something intimate about having someone unveil their secret turn-ons. She got into it.

"Softer, slave. Get it right or I will bite you—hard," she said, taking a firmer tone.

She could tell he was getting excited.

"Now, go down on me, slave."

Keis obeyed.

Then she pulled his hair. "Too fast. I'm very particular. Pay attention to what I say or be punished."

"Yes, Madame," he replied.

And with that, he came. Isabella felt victorious in her role, making him climax She liked talking dirty to men. She liked to watch the effect she had.

Isabella came to me with a question. She needed to make a decision about what she was willing to do for this love affair. She took a seat and declared with a giggle that she felt nervous sitting on the couch of a sex therapist, not that she was shy, just that it was a service she never imagined she'd employ. I warmed her up by having her tell me about how they met. Once she'd gotten comfortable, she decided to begin her story with a tale about why Keis was a great guy, before shocking me with his indecent proposal.

"My Dad has cancer. I recently found out that the treatment is no longer working. I've been expecting this time to come, but it's hard to prepare for what you're going to feel. One night last week, I had this feeling of, in my chest, I could sense the loss coming, the doom. I canceled a date with Keis. I didn't want him to see me that way. Then he shows up at my door an hour later, walks over to me, and just holds me. I started to cry and we stood there and he didn't let go. Then he drew me a bath and I sat in it while he sponged warm water over me and stroked my hair. After that I put on my pajamas and he tucked me in and read me a bedtime story. I have never had a man be so tender toward me. Ever."

Her eyes were glassy; she was still clearly moved by his nurturing.

"I'm sensing there is a 'but' to this story," I said, knowing that she had come to me for a reason.

"Yes, last night, he brought over some toys. He had cuffs and this contraption that looked like a metal cage in the shape of underwear, a chastity belt, and I thought, *Whoa, he wants me to wear that!* And then *he* put it on and he wanted me to slap his face and call him a pathetic wimp and tell him that his cock was too small to satisfy me and that he needed to be taught how to please me and that he couldn't come until I told him to. I thought I was down for anything, but I've never come across this one. I want to make him happy, but I don't know if I should do it?"

The Internet is a tableau for the sexual imagination. You can dress up like a furry rabbit or a baby in diapers, or if you like having a pie thrown in your face, there is an affirming community for you. In the modern, secular world, there is no right or wrong. Isabella believed in respecting these various forms of sexual expression, but she still needed some way to navigate this choice.

I couldn't offer her the quick and easy yes-or-no answer she wanted from me. I've always disliked the "be down for anything" advice I hear other sex therapists promoting. It's thoughtless. It puts pressure on women to do things they're not ready for and it ignores emotions. Guys should not feel entitled that their girlfriend *must* be "down." Relationships are about negotiations, not demands.

If Isabella wanted to make an informed decision about entering the world of cuckold and chastity, she needed to understand him and her own reaction. I know this kind of reflection isn't hot, but sex doesn't have a uniform significance for all—or even for one across encounters and partners. It's an existentially amorphous act. Beyond the imperative to procreate, sex has no inherent meaning. We construct the meaning. This is what makes it interesting. It's fluid, and as we change, so does the allegory of our sex.

When clients present the challenges of their sexual experiences to me, my first rule is not to judge, but I am a psychologist, so I am inclined to analyze. Psychology infiltrates sex—whether we want it to or not. One thing that has become clear to me in the practice of talking to people is that sex is rarely *just sex*.

Sex isn't just a biological act. It's a social act. People are constantly playing roles, and sexual preferences aren't inborn; they're scripts that serve a purpose. It's a constant expression and ongoing exploration of who we are. Sex is also a deeply personal act, full of unmeasured idiosyncrasies. I have my patients describe their last encounter in detail: not just their moves, but their internal dialogue and fantasy.

Fantasy is like a Rorschach test, an exposé of longings, wounds, and parts of self not actualized in everyday life. Fantasy is a container for everything we can't express: our wishes and our fears. This reverie provides a safe space for the temporary gratification of desires, revenge, or a chance to overturn that which we can't change in reality. The erotic imagination tells a story about you, your past, and who you're in the process of becoming.

Keis was into a scene loosely referred to as "cuckold and chastity." It's not uncommon; in fact, there's actually a whole online community, a cuckold "lifestyle" replete with erotica and porn, chat rooms and merchandise for sale (chastity belts, etc.). Isabella liked kinky sex but had reservations about this one. Keis sat her down and explained the role in which he'd like her to be cast. He had very specific requests. She had to be ready to make demands and to play with humiliation. He wanted to be told that his dick was pathetic and too small to please her. He wanted her to berate his body while she pleased herself with dildos bigger than him. He had some dildos in a bag that he emptied out onto the bed. They were a bit daunting in size. He also liked to watch videos on the theme, and particularly wanted to try with Isabella a scenario in which a guy called a "bull" has sex with Isabella and then cums on Keis's face or Keis is forced to pleasure the bull, all the while being called a wimp by Isabella.

Isabella was shaken. Despite her misgivings, she decided to be open minded. No stranger to edgy experiences, she'd recently had a brief stint as a girlfriend to a couple—a trend I've noticed in my practice— and with them, she attended private sex parties. Isabella agreed to watch a cuckold video. She restrained her true reaction in front of Keis and, the next day, called me. She wasn't sure how to respond. She wanted the relationship to work. She was having so much fun she could barely recall the deadness of her body while married. She didn't want to forgo the kind of chemistry that happens only a few times in one's life—but the cuckold thing freaked her out. She asked me: Do you do *anything* for the guy you care about? Should she be down for anything? If not, what are the boundaries?

These are no easy answers. There isn't a clear right or wrong path to choose. Many women are confronted with this kind of dilemma—with few tools for navigating this exciting and complex world, which offers opportunity for growth and harm.

The current state of sex culture is hard to define. In fact, I think it's in the process of defining itself or, perhaps more accurately, finding comfort without definition. Isabella wanted to be open and accepting; that's the ethos in her urban, educated world. With the endless variations of sexual tastes, it can be difficult to comprehend your reaction to it all, to find where you belong in it. I didn't want to tell her what to do; instead, I wanted to introduce her to a process for making smart decisions. Rather than blind rejection or acceptance, there are important questions. What do I want sex to mean? What am I trying to feel? How can I use sex to grow? To express myself? To be more adventurous? Less fearful? More lustful? More loving? How do I want to connect with this person? Am I causing harm to myself or others? This process of asking questions is what I like to call "conscious sexuality." Reflective, mindful, intelligent.

Isabella was clear from the beginning that she didn't want to sign up for ongoing psychotherapy. I retrieved her from the waiting room, where she was pacing impetuously. I opened the door, and she breezed past me smelling of fig and vanilla. She sat down and her shirt draped from one shoulder, revealing the amber glow of her skin. She had a mix of European and indigenous features, a proud nose, high cheekbones, round doe eyes. I gazed at her face, a symphony of two worlds; a pastiche of inharmonious features that became more enchanting with time. I told her that I was willing to consult with her for a session or two but could offer no simple solution.

"What's your reservation about playing this role he wants you to play?"

"I got turned off by him in that role. I can't stand a guy in that position. He's younger than me, so I'm already ahead of him in every sense. I make more money, have more things, etc. In the bedroom, I don't want him to be child-like."

The act of noticing is an important first step. Initial reactions can be a blur, an inchoate mass that many don't pause to disentangle because they're too blinded by their desire to please. With a few questions, the truth began to surface.

"What does it mean to you to act out a fantasy for someone?"

"My ex-husband was a college professor and he always wanted me to pretend I was a student that would do sexual favors in exchange for good grades. Either that or he wanted me to pretend I was a housemaid or a drug addict. The theme was that I was disadvantaged and I wanted something from him and had to please him to get it."

"What was the problem with that?"

"I was ambivalent. I liked role-playing in general, but at 37, I didn't like pretending I was in college and I started getting annoyed that I had to play some subservient role every single time. It started to feel like it was bad for my soul. I started to feel the effect of it in our relationship, even in my sense of self. I don't know, like I didn't feel respected and I certainly couldn't feel adored or powerful. It took me time to recover from the wounds of that relationship. Am I going down a road again, lost in someone else's preferences?"

Sexual tastes can be benign or malignant. *Fantasies* are often incongruent with identity, politically incorrect, and not necessarily related to a personality trait. *Preferences* are more repetitive, rigid, and loaded with psychological material. This doesn't mean that they're harmful, just more engrained. However, from my time working with men, I knew that sometimes the stuff they want to do is coming from a dark place. Listen to your gut.

No two couples are going to have identical turn-ons, so the process of coming together can be precarious. It's easy to lose your sense of self if you don't have a firm hold on your own style.

"Did you introduce any role-plays into the relationship with your husband?"

"Sometimes, I would make up random role-plays that would re-verse it, just to feel like I was balancing it out, but then I would sense he wasn't that into it or he would lose his erection and I got nervous and would kind of paralyze, not knowing what to say, and he would then take the lead. Eventually, we both got disconnected and over time, both of us lost interest in sex altogether. I don't want to repeat that."

The struggle here to include her desires made it too easy to shut down. Isabella needed to be clear about her own style if there was any hope of making it work with a guy like Keis—who knows exactly what he wants.

"What do you fantasize about when you masturbate?"

"Really weird stuff. It varies. This is so embarrassing to say out loud. I've never told anybody, even my husband, but I do want to tell you be-cause I'm curious about why I think about what I do. I usually fantasize about a woman giving a man a blow job."

This wasn't weird at all; in fact, words like "weird" and "normal" don't apply well to understanding fantasy. It's like saying a dream is weird or normal. I tend to explore what they feel and to ask who in the fantasy they identify with.

"Who are you in the fantasy?"

"The guy. Always the guy and I noticed that was odd. Why am I the guy? If I pretend I'm a woman or fantasize a woman being pleasured, I get turned off."

"You get turned off at yourself in a position where *you* hold the sexual command."

"Yes, why can't I get into that? Then, I don't like being in the servile role either, like I was with my ex. I got angry at myself in that position and angry at him. One time I said, 'Women have been oppressed for centuries and you're telling me that turns you on. Like, how is that sup-posed to help me to overcome the impact of that oppression?' Then I thought, *Hey, chill out, I'm an adult, this is just play, surrender to the role, it's just a game.* But I could never get into it. So, yeah, I can't do either role. I'm caught in between."

The Women on My Couch

Isabella truly was caught in between two paradigms. She was older and more successful, yet accustomed to the old hierarchy even though she hated the idea. Economically, women are now the primary breadwinners in one out of four families. Women are choosing to marry later and have children less often. We are free to be more promiscuous and can make demands for equitable pleasure. Men are more sensitive to pleasing women, which can lead to their erectile dysfunction. Numerous people have written to me complaining that men and women are all mixed up, that we need to return to the clear roles of the 1950s when "a man is a man and a woman is a woman." In reality, both genders are having to adapt to the changing roles outside the bedroom. I think in time erotic psyches will catch up to the new roles.

I found Isabella's case interesting because what turned her on was in conflict with her egalitarian ideals. What happens when the balance of power in a relationship shifts toward the woman? I've noticed a pattern in my practice of an attenuated sex drive—for the woman. I also notice anger and contempt toward men. Some pretty serious negative reactions to having more power. Don't women want to enjoy this position? She could dominate a man, celebrate her conquest. Why doesn't this work? I can think of a few reasons. First of all, women aren't conditioned to find men who are dependent, incompetent, or less intelligent to be sexy (as men are with women). Sometimes, there is a mother–child dynamic happening that isn't very appealing. Perhaps she is doing his laundry, packing his lunch, tying his shoelaces. Women resent this, even when they're complicit.

I left my office to get a cup of coffee on Sunset Boulevard, which is no place for strolling and thinking. Just out the front door and I see a drag queen in sequined shorts doing a downward dog—likely preparing for a show in a neighboring gay bar. There were cars, motorcycles, homeless people, Mexican cowboys, gals in vintage dresses, and a couple elder Armenian ladies ambling about. In the midst of such diversity, I became more aware that everyone has a story, and this story is part of their Eros. Isabella's mind was shaped by two worlds. Her parents were immigrants from El Salvador and hard-core Catholics. Raised in L.A.,

Isabella wanted to be like the California blonde bombshells. She was interested in tattoos and feminism. She worked hard to extricate herself from her parents' stuffy morality. It was a fierce fight that, at times, got physical. It was a strict authoritarian family, an organized structure of rules and chores with no democracy. As a teenager, she became rebellious; her entire personality became organized around being the opposite of her parents. And all her choices in men reflected this imperative.

I turned down a side street and found a quiet block, the kind of respite one can't find in New York. I thought about how life experiences form an erotic map. Specifications for attraction begin early. The associations we make to touch and intimacy with our parents—all the way back to our preverbal period—are actually imprinted in our brain. Freud was right: mom was your first sex object. Even if she was abusive, you probably still loved her, and that is the very sort of ambivalence that explains our sexual tastes—dualities and contradictions. This history impacts masturbation fantasies, actual bedroom behavior, and what attracts you to someone.

Children and adolescents often eroticize their pain. Traumatic experiences, such as physical abuse or rejection by the person you have a crush on, can become sexualized and acted out in ways that symbolically re-create the trauma. Many preferences can be traced to puberty. Were we rejected, popular, bullied, sexualized by adults? How did we handle competition from the opposite sex? From our same-sex parent? How did our first sexual experience go? These situations affect how we approach love and sex. They determine how hungry we are for attention, validation, affection, and even masochism or sadism. When these desires lead to problematic patterns, this is "unconscious sexuality."

Isabella's first husband, Mark, was domineering. Yes, she made that cliché move of marrying one's father. She rebelled against Mark—but she liked it. She started fights and then had great sex. That worked for both of them until he lost his job, and his self-esteem took a hit. Without an authority figure to sexualize, she lost interest in sex.

Isabella was turned on by alpha men—and she wanted to fight with them. The parent–child relationship is certainly not egalitarian.

Therefore, our first and most formative relationship is hierarchical, and we all start at the bottom. The interactions around this power differential shape our personal relationship with power.

Now that Isabella's father was dying, she was no longer interested in being the woman who rebels against men. She longed, for softness, not friction. That old pattern that was once so strong, that once filled her sexual adventures, was loosening its grip. She saw that her desires were actually quite fleeting. I saw this as a good thing, that her erotic psyche adapted to her life. She wasn't totally stuck. Preferences become a problem when the erotic repertoire is fixated, narrow, and rigid. Some women or men *must* be in control or *must* have a dominant partner. But modern American couples don't exist in a fixed hierarchy.

Keis clearly had his own history and desires. And Isabella, deep down, wanted something totally different from sex. Could they compromise?

Isabella and I were trying to take the route of conscious sexuality, so we began to apply the process of questioning. *What did she need now?* She seemed to be searching for a sense of balance.

"Is it doing harm to him?" she asked. "I can't tell. I wonder if he was abused or something?"

I wanted to refrain from armchair analyzing Keis, so I continued to redirect Isabella toward understanding herself.

"Is it doing harm to you?"

"No, but it doesn't fit what I'm looking for."

"What do you most want from sex right now, Isabella?"

"I'm grieving my father already, I'm kind of raw right now. What I really want most is more of that moment in the bathtub, when he was stroking my head. That's what I want right now. I wanted to walk the streets and hold hands and to go back home and tear each other's clothes off…and then have regular sex."

"So, then, are you getting the connection you want?"

"No."

"Is it OK if you don't get it every time?"

"I guess, if I get it a lot of the time."

Isabella wanted passionate nights with her eccentric musician lover to help her hold on to the beauty of life as she was faced with the realities of death. She didn't want to marry this guy or even get serious.

"I don't want to call him a wimp. I just want to smell his skin and write poems on his body with markers, to feel his young, brazen energy move inside me."

Isabella made her decision quickly. After realizing that her past relationships were driven by reactions to her strict parents or a heedless desire to please her husband, she wondered where her life would have led if she hadn't been so reactive to them. She declared that it was time for a path of self-determination. She was old enough to know that the most charming, razzle-dazzle road, festooned with lights and laughs, is not always the right path. It was only mirage, a high-voltage rabbit hole. She didn't want to unravel all the rebuilding she'd done after her divorce. She decided to break it off with Keis before getting more involved. She did it over the phone. She said if she'd seen him in person, there'd be no way she could resist the pull of the chemical reaction between them. That call was heartrending for her.

I suggested that she stay in therapy. She just said no to something, and now she needed something to say yes to. We began to explore what direction she could go next. I introduced her to an idea that is gaining popularity among women who are looking to define a sexuality on their own terms: Taoist practices.

Taoism also offers an answer to the modern question: Can we have both equality and desire? Modern research says no, that power imbalance is a universal turn-on. And in modern times, they're right. But it hasn't always been that way. Again, history offers another story. One of the most richly sensual periods, one famed for its "Love Masters" and multi-orgasmic women, didn't focus on role-plays or hierarchies. The time was 2,000 years ago. The place was China. A time of silk robes, orchid-scented bedrooms, and making love on silk-netted beds in the soft light of a lantern or outdoors in the spring when the cherry trees were in bloom. The famous Tao of Love texts and art came from an era of lush feminine sensuality, a time also known for its relative gender equality.

The Women on My Couch

The Tao of Love texts offer a simplicity that seemed just right for where Isabella was in her life. Sex was seen as medicinal, considered nourishing and replenishing. I find the Taoist perspective of desire to be useful when couples come in with differences like Isabella and Keis had. Sometimes, they're so overwhelmed by the differences in their preferences that it's helpful to reset by returning to the basics of sex. By letting go of all the mentalizations of fantasy and identity and neuroses, they can come back to the rudiments of pleasure: the senses.

While Western researchers are still debating over the exact location of the G-spot, a host of sex coaches out there are orgasming away with Taoist-derived techniques that they teach at retreats and conferences and in one-on-one coaching. Sex is trumpeted as everything from the medicinal to the magical. Daily orgasms, orgasmic meditation, and even swallowing cum are said to heal depression, enhance creativity, and fatten your bank account. Some websites read like a pep rally for sex, with slogans for "tapping into your power," intimating that the womb contains a dormant source of power that, once awakened, will not only transform your life but also the entire world. These websites are heavy on the sales pitch, exalting sex as some panacea—about which I'm skeptical—but these experts do seem to genuinely exude the sex appeal, charm, and confidence promised by their exercises.

I decided to check out one of these workshops before I considered referring my clients. The workshop I attended was billed as a teaching on ancient feminine arts. Right away, the instructor, a petite woman with a soft voice yet commanding presence, had us standing up doing a series of hip rocking, rolling, and other fluid movements.

We were in a living room in suburban Los Angeles rocking our collective hips to sitar music, loosening the pelvis, a part of the body that gets constricted in the daily life of a modern woman. "We must wake up the womb," she instructed, which is the center of sexual energy—implying that women are the source of lust, not just the object of it. Further, she taught that sexual energy is connected to a larger, universal energy responsible for all creative action, including the force that makes plants grow, waves rise, wounds heal, babies germinate, and creative ideas flow. All women have the ability to tap in.

Techniques for "awakening the feminine" were varied. We were instructed to close our eyes and gently touch each part of our body with an attitude of regard, silently whispering affirmations of love to each. Because sexual energy is thought to grow in a relaxed state, we practiced breathing slowly. We walked around the room, moving each part of our body, slowly and consciously.

The ancient belief is that once a woman awakens her womb, an innate intelligence begins to operate, causing her to emanate charm, sex appeal, and passion. "Beauty is an energy," said the instructor, "not one's physical dimensions." Beauty isn't about what you're wearing. It's that spark in your soul that inspired you to decorate yourself.

I totally loved this woman. She wore colorful clothing and ethnic jewelry and just radiated sensuality. I left thinking I may have found my favorite Aphrodite. Small groups are sprouting up around the globe, and importantly, they're offering a new narrative about female libido. "Sex isn't something you give away," she said. "Sex is an act that brings replenishment. Your sexual energy is your power." Sexual desire is not some irrelevant titillation but an important life force, a moment of connecting to a force greater than oneself. I believe these coaches *can* change the psychological and physical patterns that keep women from developing sexually.

I referred Isabella to a local Taoist center, and she began to try out the practices. In session, I asked for her reaction.

"I feel calm, feminine. By the way, I met a guy at a Taoist retreat. We had sex and it was sweet and tender. He was all about pleasing me. It was good, but…I don't know, maybe he's too nice," she said, scrunching up her nose.

I was suspicious of the "too nice" excuse.

"You don't want a guy to be nice to you?"

"He's trying so hard to make me happy, he's apprehensive about his every move. I wish he'd relax."

Nice guys do have it tough. But the problem isn't their being a good guy. The real problems are the behaviors we mistakenly label as "nice":

pleasing, ingratiating, and lack of decisiveness, confidence, or leadership. This isn't nice; it's insecurity.

Taoism was all about the action of opposing essences, Yin and Yang. Isabella wanted to feel soft in contrast to his strength. Yet, in Taoism men were also trained in sophisticated sexual skills, including the ability to love. Imagine a system teaching men to measure their masculinity not by conquest but by their capacity to love.

"I like Taoism, but it's not enough to turn me on."

I wasn't sure if she was capable of receiving the nurturing she claimed she wanted or if she needed the excitement of rebelling against pushy men. Many of my clients fetishize bad boys or alpha males or Christian Grey types, but in reality, most guys aren't edgy, and it's not a man's job to make your life exciting. I kept her focused on what she is responsible for—herself.

"Have the mediation practices helped to turn you on?"

"Yes, they work! I did the vagina breathing one."

This meditation involves simply resting attention on the clitoris and breathing. I was skeptical when I first read about this exercise, but I decided to give it ten minutes of my time without trying too hard. I was startled at the sensation. I felt a moderate throbbing without even touching myself. I imagined this was what a horny guy feels. The achy, lusty sensation is further heightened with a little hip rocking and Kegel squeezes. I practiced this vagina breathing meditation, over and over, starting from different mood states, and continued to get the same result in varying degrees of intensity. This experiential learning was important to me because there's so much focus in psychology on whether women even have a sex drive, and it was as if my body had shared its truth, that sexual energy is right there, sitting dormant in my pelvis, a subtle energy always present, waiting to reveal itself.

Taoist techniques have none of the pizzaz and dopamine rush that one would get from porn or a whip or a little dirty talk. It's not easy gratification; it's a slow but effective burn. Most modern women demand more intensity, but I couldn't help but wonder what living in China 2,000 years ago was like for a woman's desire. Human bodies and various sex acts were widely exalted in art and literature in an ever present poetic expression of life. It was a period of openness; there was no religion censuring sex, thus no guilt and no need to eroticize what is dirty and forbidden because those ideas did not exist to react to. Sadomasochism is reputed to have been absent. Pejorative sexual language didn't exist as it does today; genital terminology was couched in poetic language, such as the jade stem for the penis and, for the vagina: the jade gate, the golden lotus, the open peony blossom, and the receptive vase. Did all of this create an atmosphere for an easy experience of desire? Did they have to try as hard as we do?

I'd started dating an experienced outdoorsman. The kind of guy who goes on ten-day solo backpacking trips in the Sierra Nevada, a fisherman who could catch a trout and clean, cook, and feed it to me right there on the bank of a remote mountain lake. A nature guide sounded exotic after my time in New York. He took me camping at Big Sur. At 1 a.m., we went to a hot spring pool nestled in the side of a cliff overlooking the ocean. Lounging in the steaming water, nude, under the moon, hearing the crash of the waves hundreds of feet below, a new consciousness began to emerge for me.

Inspired ancient erotic Chinese poems placed sex in relation to the natural world: bodies and trees, embraces and seasons, longing and flowers were inseparable. I wanted my naked skin to feel the warm sun or a cool creek, to brush the grass of a meadow. We went on more trips, high into the Sierra Nevada and Rocky Mountains, into old forests with crystalline lakes and gentle ponds. In the grandeur of being deep in the outdoors, I began to lose my self-consciousness. I experienced myself as part of a bigger natural world, and all of my constructed meaning about sex, various sex acts, and bodies faded out and I became just a woman on a riverbank. My hang-ups seemed trifling in this setting. Somehow the sexual current of the wild gave me permission to let go, to dive into pleasure without reservation, and it finally felt like a natural right.

The Women on My Couch

Isabella stayed in therapy for a while longer than she anticipated. Most of our time together centered on her father's illness and her desire to live life to the fullest. She practiced Taoism regularly and continued to date. When I last saw her, she was still single and concerned she wouldn't find someone. But she was equipped with the ability to make wise decisions and felt more solid about her sexual style.

In Taoism, there is no scarcity of sexual energy—nor is it necessary to find a specific person to incite the libido. It's right there, at the core of our being. The idea is to turn inward and connect. Desire can be sought for its own sake. The purpose is to radiate, to create, to attract—a way of being that is very different from the common ego-based sexual motivation that causes suffering. Western perception is that only the sexy people are in a position of power, and we worry about feeling foolish if our advances aren't returned. Wanting is weak; desire is feared.

For Taoists, desire is power.

Cassie

My Manhattan private practice was filled with bankers and businessmen. In Hollywood, my office began to fill up with people in "The Business." My new clients were actors, directors, producers, writers—and people who wanted to be those things. In coffee shops, restaurants, and lounges, Hollywood fizzes and crackles with discussions about character arcs, plot development, and the hero's quest. The hum of their passion is contagious. Countless people I meet, in all manner of professions, are working on a script.

I like the Hollywood hopefuls because they're brave. A theme in therapy here is living with uncertainty. Despite talent, hard work, and beauty, their fate is determined by meeting the right people, timing, and luck. It's hard to surrender your life to those forces—especially when you graduated from college with a 4.0, like my client Cassie. She did have something to lose. Yet her romantic hope was palpable. Every stranger held possibility: a ticket into an agency, an audition, or a successful boyfriend.

Cassie didn't have a problem finding men. Her inbox on OkCupid was so full, she didn't even have time to read all the messages. She spent at least five nights a week on dates, the other two devoted to preparations for upcoming dates: getting her nails done, buying new dresses, touching up blonde roots—all symbols of her unyielding hope that eventually she would find him. The One. Cassie wasn't inclined to sit and wait haplessly for destiny to decide upon the timing. She would manifest him now. A vision board, full of magazine cutouts of men, sat atop her bedroom dresser.

The Women on My Couch

"He has to be in my age range—no older creepers. No guys with bare-chested pics (because I don't need to see you naked just yet) and definitely, no guys who have other women hanging on them in their pics (duh). What I want is simple: a classy guy, with good manners who is successful. I love, love guys in suits: bankers, real estate developers, lawyers. Ahh, a well-dressed man." She smiled and looked up dreamily.

"This might be too much to ask, but you get what you ask for, so he does have to be good looking," she said as she tossed her hair.

Cassie had a sunny composition, and at first impression, I was charmed. For the past seven years, no relationship had lasted more than a few months. My task was to help her understand why, in all that time, she never felt that fated-by-the-gods kind of attraction. Nor did the guys she met. She could attract men, but she couldn't keep them.

"I don't get it, I'm a catch."

Cassie pulled out her iPhone to show me her dating site profile.

"What's wrong with this profile?"

Her lead picture was a professional headshot. She had a polished smile, a button nose smattered with freckles, and hair the color of wheat. Other photos included the cliché mountaintop in Peru shots that are supposed to demonstrate how adventurous one is. Then, there was a slew of seductive selfies to show her tarty side, tumbled hair, head down, and eyes up, with a convincing come-hither stare. The text on her profile was brief and generic, "because guys don't read it, they just look at the pics."

Her profile certainly showcased her marketing skills. She was the girl next door and sexy and willing to backpack. One of my friends joked about this contrived advertising and said a realist snapshot would include her in a wedding dress, walking down the street pushing an empty baby stroller, with a caption saying "OK, I'm ready now."

Upon entering my office for the first time, Cassie's greeting was formal, with the affected confidence and cheer one often finds in a sales professional. She sat down on the couch, legs crossed and hands folded across her lap like she was at a junior league luncheon—this very self-contained presentation in stark contrast to the wild abandon she portrayed in her series of selfies. She flashed a wide, very white smile and made direct eye contact as she began to tell me her dating history.

"Maybe its technology or L.A. Men get the sense of limitless possibility—and it's true, the harvest season for hot young actresses has no end. Why should they settle? But most people do eventually get married, so maybe there is something wrong with me. Obviously, I can't see what it is."

I filed away the judgment that something was "wrong" with her.

"Sounds like you have a strong sense that dating is a competition."

"It makes me crazy. Yes, if you're online, you're aware of it. It takes all the romance out, we're like a bunch of cattle at an auction. But I play the game. I think my looks are above average and I do everything possible to better them. I lift weights. I get my hair done, I have Latisse for my eyelashes, a tiny bit of Botox around my eyes because I smile a lot, teeth whitened. I take care of all of the details."

This beauty regimen may sound like an L.A. cliché, but it's a reality for sometimes-working actresses like Cassie who live in Santa Monica, a town that thinks it's a giant outdoor gymnasium, with a few regular pedestrians milling about, always in the way of the runners. Every inch of green space is taken up by personal trainers barking orders at ripped people. Elderly folks complain to the city council that they can't relax with people doing jumping jacks in all directions.

I noted that image was her primary focus, not common interests or emotional qualities. Rather than being a mystery that unfolds over the course of dating, so much of one's self-image has to be prepackaged and placed among others in a marketplace. Cassie seemed to understand herself in terms of what is salable, and she was willing to adjust her appearance—her brand—the basis of what is known to sell. She said she was playing the game, but did she know the difference between her online profile and who she actually was?

"You talk about your body like it's a product to be marketed."

She looked me up and down, as if appraising my appearance, perhaps returning a judgment.

"Call it self-objectification if you want, but it feels good," she said, sounding blasé—a cool affectation I found unique to L.A.

She didn't like my comment. And in truth, it was my own projection, not an accurate follow of her true concern.

"I see that you're not married," she said, intoning that, obviously, something was amiss with me. It stung, but I wasn't falling for it.

I wasn't going to tell Cassie, but I was also dating online. And she had much more dating experience. After a six-year relationship, I was new to online dating. Unlike Cassie, I wasn't in search of a relationship, so I didn't have her urgency. As an experiment, I'd decided to go out with everyone who asked me, regardless of whether he was my type, thinking I was opening myself to new possibilities. I'd written in my profile text that I officially had no requirements, that I was dating without parameters—to which a bunch of guys wrote back, "Wow, you said parameters."

This is what my experiment yielded: a man whose legal name was King, who lived in a house patterned after the Palace of Versailles, literally with a gold-gilded throne at his kitchen table. He rejected me for wearing cheap shoes. I went out with a guy who liked to apply women's lip gloss several times an hour and who told me I should put on a thicker layer of eyeliner and lose a little belly fat. I went out with a movie "producer" before I was warned that meant he probably sat at home all day in his boxers writing scripts. I also went out with a military interrogator and an older philanthropist with a foot fetish.

Once in a while, I'll share my personal experiences with a client, but most of the time, they have no clue what's happening in my life or if I've been through the same kinds of experiences or, like Cassie, I'm in a similar place. I could identify with the pressure Cassie felt to market her image; the Internet lends itself to rapid assessments, and she was simply trying to adapt to the norms of modern dating.

After work I'd scan, perhaps the same, pixelated faces. Men posted photos of European travel, poses with puppies or babies, shirtless pics, and action shots of their exercise routine: running, hiking, biking. Perfect bodies, exciting international trips, wild nightlife—is this what makes a relationship? Of course not, but it is effective ad copy. We seek our reflection in all the shiny objects that surround us, our cars, clothes, degrees. And like the sparkling imagery, our stylized lives dilute who we really are. We're all chasing an ideal self, sometimes to destruction.

On a weekend trip to Palm Springs, I walked down the main drag to see the city's proud new art installation. A twenty-six-foot Marilyn Monroe, towering above the buildings like King Kong. Her two legs open, straddling the side walk, tourists clinging to her calves under her flared skirt. Her giant head was thrown back, her face smiling. Thinking of Cassie, and the whole online dating scene, I reflected on the importance of image, Marilyn's in particular—she, our supreme female representation, America's Aphrodite—and what it means to our society. The sheer size of that statue demonstrates how her figure lords over us, her adorants.

One of the biggest surprises in my historical perusing was in the transcripts from Marilyn Monroe's psychoanalyst (which are public record as a result of the investigation following her death). In between therapy sessions, Marilyn would talk, or "free associate," into a tape recorder at home or on the road, and then she'd send the tape to her analyst, Dr. Ralph Greenson. Right before her death, one of the main issues addressed in therapy was an inability to have an orgasm.

"What I told you is true when I first became your patient. I had never had an orgasm...."

When I read this quote, I literally froze for a moment, aghast and disoriented. It was like finding out that Santa isn't real. Marilyn Monroe is the most famous *sex* symbol of the twentieth century. She also confessed:

"I would win overwhelmingly if the Academy gave an Oscar for faking orgasms. I have done some of my best acting convincing my partners I was in the throes of ecstasy."

I marveled at the thought of how many men must have climaxed to her image. Yet *she* wasn't having orgasms? Our Goddess of Eros had been exposed as an ordinary woman still searching for her clit. This incongruity represents where many women are today in their sexual development: straddled between an image and the real woman.

Marilyn lamented, "A sex symbol becomes a thing; I hate being a thing," but also said, "I don't mind being burdened with being glamorous and sexual." Though I love this line and am totally going to use it as an affirmation, there's an obvious contrast between the command she had over her appeal and the faking of orgasms. She certainly enjoyed her seductive abilities, but only at the end of her life did she learn that being *sexy* is not the same thing as being *sexual*.

Marilyn Monroe lived as her mask, a mirror of projected desires. And why would she want to live as her authentic self? The rewards for remaining an object of fantasy were great. Worldwide adoration, to be exact. Women today are also confronted with the same standards of sexiness and we make many small choices about adhering to expectations or following our instincts—and we're only seeking the adoration of one man (or possibly a few more than that).

Getting lost in the pursuit of validation of beauty is the same trap that disconnects everyday women from their bodies. *Adoration is an emotional need, not sexual energy.* When talk therapy failed, Marilyn's analyst instructed her to simply masturbate. And, finally, in her mid-thirties, Marilyn had her first orgasm. The transcript reads:

"Bless you, Doctor. What you say is gospel to me. By now I've had lots of orgasms. Not only one, but two and three with a man who takes his time….I never cried so hard as I did after my first orgasm. It was because of the years I had…never had an orgasm. What wasted years."

Assigning masturbation was a simple and brilliant intervention. Her success was about more than an orgasm; the connection to body is a means of self-connection. True sexiness is to inhabit one's body and connect to that internal sexual current. Men can sense this.

Cassie needed to learn this lesson. I wished she had some of Marilyn's ambivalence—or insight. When Cassie goes on a date, the man sitting across the dinner table casually chatting about his dog is unconsciously seeing more than just her bright smile and lush eyelashes; the emotional center in his brain is scanning hers. The term for this in neuroscience is *limbic resonance*—named after the limbic system, the regulatory structure of the emotions in the brain. People don't just see each other, we feel each other as well. We can *feel* the truth. And our physiology responds by adapting to that truth. So, if Cassie feels her own sexual desire, he will sense it. However, on first dates, it's usually hidden behind a wall of anxiety and self-consciousness. Limbic resonance can revolutionize the way we think about attractiveness and seduction. Moving beyond the mirage of appearance, we can learn to become more sexually embodied. To cultivate our sexual desire from within—as a source of magnetism. Cassie looked the part, but did she have a palpable sexual energy?

At thirty-three, Cassie had clearly sowed her oats with men and was also well traveled. The restlessness of wanting to explore every inch of the planet had begun to settle and she could finally consider children without feeling like she was going to miss out or give up too much. As for her career, although she spent more time driving for Uber than she did acting, her faith crested after a recent part in a small, one-time role for a hit TV show and she'd booked a commercial. She had a solid social network and didn't view herself as needy or desperate. Just ready.

"What do *you* sense is missing on your dates?" I asked her.

"A connection that clicks. I went on a date last night and when he walked me to my car, there was an awkward moment. He was telling me a funny story about his dog when we got to the car, and then I paused, looked him in the eye to make a connection, and he kissed me…but it was brief and we each said good night and that was it. I haven't heard from him today. It seems like the kiss is a litmus test, if it doesn't go well, you're not gonna get a callback. So, I've been trying to replay in my mind what went wrong. Maybe it was because we were talking about our pets and you can't just transition from that into a hot kiss."

The end-of-date first kiss can feel like the forced gaiety of Christmas or New Year's: it's tough to manufacture happiness or a hot kiss simply because an occasion calls for it. I wondered what else there was to her besides the seemingly implacable positive demeanor.

"Give me one word to describe the feel of the date."

The Women on My Couch

"Pleasant."

Perhaps that was the problem.

"Would you want to go out with him again?"

"No, but I still check my phone all day."

"You just want him to want you?"

Those anxious moments of waiting—to find out if you've been chosen, if you're desired—can be so breath bating for people that they mistake it for actually liking the person. Anybody on dating websites knows they are just one in a sea of people, yet secretly they hope they stand out from the rest of the ruck. Nobody wants to realize after an evening of opening yourself, sharing your world or even your body, that in fact, to him, you were just another inconsequential face, a throwaway evening.

As I sat listening to her story, I tried to feel her. It was like trying to feel the soul of my desk. She was candid and open, but when she told a story it was filled with facts and tons of irrelevant details, which I'm sparing here. A wall of words—the name of the restaurant, the route they took to get there, a side story about the owner of the restaurant whom she'd known in middle school—almost put me into a coma. When clients do this, I typically put my hand up and say, "Pause." But Cassie chatted like a sorority girl on Ritalin, and I was having a hard time finding an opening. Finally, I interrupted her.

"I'm going to stop you. I'm noticing that I feel disconnected and I want to point that out to see if it helps us understand what happens on dates."

"You do? What am I doing?"

"I feel shut out by the length of your story."

"I thought the more you talk in therapy the better."

"For me or for you?"

"I guess I thought that's what you want?"

"Let's gauge it by how *you* feel."

She paused in a confused tension.

"I'm not sure if I'm getting anywhere," she said apprehensively, as if waiting for my disapproval.

58

"I'm glad we're discovering this. If you'd keep following what you imagine I want—then we're not getting to the heart of your issue. Does this happen when you're with men—do you try to be what they want?"

"I'm kind of like water. I can be very attuned to a guy's personality and flow with it. I know I'm supposed to ask questions and listen—and that I should share about myself as well. I thought that was a good social skill?"

Cassie was very formal, polite and pleasing as well. She had learned good social skills; she just wasn't executing them effectively.

"So, your proclivity is to accommodate what the other person is looking for?"

"In my family, nobody ever disagrees or challenges or asks provocative questions. We sit at the dinner table on Thanksgiving, the entire extended family, and we talk about the food, and kids and dogs. That's it. Everybody has the exact same personality. If our collective personality had a color, it would be taupe."

"Do you like the color taupe?" I smiled.

"It's sooo boring. But I don't challenge it. I'm one of them. I dress like them, talk like them—but that's who I am. I don't dislike it."

"What would happen if you shook it up and talked about a controversial issue?"

"If somebody actually expresses an opinion, say, about politics or religion, that is known to be different than the rest of my family, everyone will be like, *wow—that's so weird.*"

"The entire family has the same political point of view?"

"Yes, and they feel superior about it. The other side—all idiots."

"So, the lesson you've learned is to blend into the room."

"Yes."

"I want to understand the consequence of that. Will you try an experiment for me?"

"Yes."

I was really appreciating her candor in this moment. I decided to keep going deeper.

"Let's give voice to the rules you learned in your family. Have the voice sound like a dictator. What would it say?"

"Don't stand out."

"Continue. Let the voice sound very demanding."

"Do not be different."

"What else?"

"Do not cry. Do not show weakness. Do not fail. Show your best self or nothing at all."

"Or what?"

"Or you are an idiot."

I was deep in the voice of her resistance, that shield preventing all of her from joining me, from joining men. It's important to draw the resistance out of its hidden control room, into the light, where it loses power.

"OK, let's pause there. How does this sound to you?"

"Crazy. Like you can't have any real emotions." She laughed at the absurdity.

"What happens to your secret feelings?"

"I try not to feel them."

I tilted my head, feeling sad for her, for the labor of having to suppress.

"They aren't pretty like the rest of you."

She paused and looked at the floor.

"Right."

"What if I think they're pretty? Can I see those parts of you?" I asked gently.

"I don't know." She kept her head down, her body answering the question.

She seemed to use prettiness as a form of denial. A defense against experiencing anything real. She was all lovely and competent, and I imagined her living room was all white and clean, with fresh pink tulips in a jar.

"Is there a part of you that wants to be free?"

"I don't know. I'm scared."

"I can't really feel you. No emotions. No vulnerability," I said softly.

"I don't know if I can change that. Maybe this is my personality," she said, returning to eye contact.

"Being inauthentic is not a personality trait. It's a bad habit. Let's set a new rule for this room. No polite façades. Let's be ourselves. You can curse, say your opinions, disagree, and be irrational. I'll welcome that."

"How will this help me on a date?"

"If a guy can't feel you, how is he going to connect to you emotionally?"

She paused and looked down and then back up at me with moist eyes. I leaned forward to meet the intensity I could now feel.

"I want to open myself to you. I do, I want it so bad, to really share everything. The idea of that makes me want to cry."

In that moment, I remembered what it is to be a therapy client. The wish to give oneself over to the all-knowing and all-loving therapist; the surrender in revealing that tender longing to be nurtured—even though one's aware that this gift is given to a person who is being paid, a person with many clients. Many times my clients have compared me to a prostitute for this work. And, of course, that thought assumes I'm an emotional mercenary. But, in truth, I care deeply, and even more, when they finally allow me access to their inner sanctum.

Cassie's obsession with image caused more than just relationship problems. She was also in debt financially. She'd even written me two bad checks. I had to confront her and learned that she grew up in a wealthy suburb of Chicago and her parents divorced when she was a toddler. Her mother kept the house and the kids, and as a result, they grew up poor in a rich neighborhood. It was important to her mother that they kept up the appearance of having money. There were three sisters, all competitive; Cassie had perfect grades, one sister had an eating disorder, and the other compulsively stole her sisters' boyfriends.

I'd been looking for my modern-day Aphrodite, a figure to invoke lust, when I came across a website that had won the "sexiest blog" award for several years running. On the front page was pictured a middle-aged woman—not as an idol but as a raw and real woman—who'd posted a series of photographs, poems, and erotic stories, all created to portray the essence of a woman's desire. Her pseudonym is Cheeky Minx, and I began to prescribe her blog *Love Hate Sex Cake* to my clients.

Always interested in bridging the gap between psychology and erotic artists, I decided to contact Cheeky Minx. Psychologists spend too much time researching the problem and not enough time examining women at their hottest. I emailed Cheeky Minx and landed an interview. Here is a great quote about what inspired her to write the blog:

> The relationship I have with that body, with the body, mind and heart nexus, is key. As I've grown older, I've become more open and infinitely kinder to myself; I've tried to resist listening to the critical voices and judgments about my imperfections. I try and do, and often succeed. And just as often fail. But in those moments, I submerge myself in both the sexual and non-sexual as a way to reclaim myself and my desire: I walk along the river near my home; I dance around my sitting room with joy; I laugh loudly; I cry and scream and sing in the shower; I flirt with the glorious men in my life, both up close and online; I free my cheekiness; I indulge in sensual touch and carnal fucking and intense lovemaking; I treat myself and him to the filthiest phone sex we can conjure and conceive; I hone my critical mind; I give my heart and love to the deserving; I read and devour erotic literature and imagery; I masturbate—a lot; I dress myself in exquisite lingerie, in the clothes that leave me feeling dazzling; I gaze at my nakedness in the mirror; I share my experiences with like-minded and generous people; I take to the camera once again, shooting this exhibitionist in glowing light, at the times of day I feel at my best (or even worst), sensual, sexy, carnal, emotional. In the end, the photographs are also reminders for me—that I am a desirable and passionate woman, flaws and foibles and all.

Cassie was missing the cultivation of an inner appeal that could radiate outward. Cheeky is a figure one may find objectively beautiful, or not, yet that somehow seems irrelevant as she captures *the whole of a woman's sexual aliveness*—from earthy desires to careful tending of her self-esteem. By turning inward, she rescues the gaze from the adoring public and returns it to the woman. This is what a woman looks like in the absence of self-conscious posing, an ego dissolved in the stream of lust. She is all electricity, and I, the reader, was incited. I had found an Aphrodite.

Cassie cried when she read Cheeky's blog. What Cassie lacked, and she didn't even know it, was for someone to see who she was under her appearance, to shine a light on her ideas, wishes, fears—and to cherish it all. She learned so young to shut down the impulse to bring her "self" to her mother, to say, *Here I am—this is me*. She didn't even realize it needed attention until I'd made an effort to find her. The word for this in psychology is "mirroring": the act of reflecting back the client's internal state, and it is so powerful it drives people to love or, in Cassie's case, to tears.

The day of our next session, I'd arrived at my office early to do treatment planning when a noise, like the wailing cry of a man followed by a tossed salad of words—utter nonsense at high volume—sent me outside to see if I could offer assistance to what I assumed was a mentally ill man in the building, not an unrealistic scenario in my neighborhood. In the hallway were a sign that read AUDITIONS and several men sitting on chairs. This was when I learned that I was sharing office space with a production company—actually, three of them. They kindly agreed to keep the simulations of mental illness down so I could do some real therapy. Cassie walked into the building, her eyes gleaming as she glanced over at the row of handsome men trying to look disheveled. She'd met a new guy.

"His name is Cole. We went to brunch and talked all morning. I moved my chair close to him and put my head on his shoulder, and then I kissed him—I've never done that before. Finally, I felt a spark! He invited me to his lake house in Big Bear. The house was gorgeous, like a Swiss chalet, high ceilings, and stone-walled fireplace. He walked me around the grounds—we crossed a grassy meadow and up a hill where there was a lake, which was crystal clear in the sun. We walked out on the dock and he jumped in with his clothes on and so did I. He took his clothes off and threw them up on the dock. I took mine off and then swam to the other side of the lake and lay down on the grassy bank in the sun. He followed and we lay there in the sun kissing. It was a magical day. I stayed over there all weekend. He didn't want me to leave that night so he took me out to buy clothes for the weekend. I cooked for him, we laid around outside, it was glorious. He's inviting me to go away for a weekend in New Orleans!"

She was less wooden than in previous sessions. She had that insuppressible grin as she rhapsodized about her weekend.

"You seem ecstatic."

"Ahhhhh, finally, finally, I think I've found him. I know I'm getting carried away, but I could see myself with this guy." She bit her lip, suppressing her unbridled excitement.

"Let your fantasies about him get carried away for a minute. Where does your mind go?"

"Oh my God, spending every summer at that lake house. Winters at his condo downtown. Travel. Marriage, babies." She laughed. "Am I crazy to have all these fantasies after one weekend?"

"Your wishes are important. Continue."

"I imagine I'm proud to be his wife. He's very successful, so I imagine I could quit working for a while and just enjoy being a new mom. Little walks down sunny streets pushing a stroller. Having a nanny. Lunching with my friends. I would feel safe with him. A lady of leisure."

Cassie was elated, but I was dubious. Did she meet the man she's been waiting for or was this a Cinderella fantasy? Not only do women's self-images get altered in the dating process but so does our image of men. Dating is a time of uncertainty—and where there is ambiguity, people project. The same wishes have echoed from many of the women on my couch; wishes for the hero, the warrior, the knight in shining armor archetypes to rescue and save us. We create idols, a "love object." Yes, this is objectification, and it's unfair to men.

Cassie's father had left her mother for another woman, started another family, and wasn't a consistent financial provider, leaving Cassie with a hope that her Dad would return as her Knight in Shining Armor. She tried to get his attention but rarely succeeded, nor did her father ever see that longing in her. She wasn't mirrored by him, and her parade of men were all substitute mirrors, providing validation of her desirability.

When Cassie went out with her girlfriends to look for guys, they'd go to Beverly Hills, hoping to meet some wealthy studio executive, or to Sunset Boulevard in Hollywood, hoping to meet a celebrity. They never found what they were looking for; instead, they found themselves in a sea of women in tight dresses and high heels, fighting each other by the end of the night.

Like the other aspiring actors, directors, and writers I see on a daily basis, Cassie's career was fraught with uncertainty: no biweekly paycheck, no linear career trajectory, and no meritocracy. Cassie dropped out of a college in the Midwest to pursue her passion—and the threat of wasted potential constantly loomed as she watched her friends back home build families and wealth. Her mother judged from afar as she reported on small parts in various web series that failed to impress. And The Business drops just enough crumbs, a gig here and there, to keep one hoping. Like Cassie, everyone has a way of coping: New Age spirituality (just "vision" the success and it will come) or amped-up ambition (if I just lock myself in my room for the next three months, the next script I write will hit the jackpot) or landing one of L.A.'s many rich men as a husband. Cassie didn't want to acknowledge that she teetered on despair. She wanted to believe something great was about to happen. So, she focused on her body, on men, and on her next audition. She wished that the world would discover she was special or that a Prince Charming would take her away to his palace in the Hollywood Hills.

As a psychotherapist, I spend a lot of time untangling love from illusion. Dreams of being bigger, better, more desirable are very much a part of the American psyche. Fantasy inspires us toward our best selves—and can drive us to destruction as well. Even I had to address the question in my own life. The idealized image I sought was still shuffling off its metaphorical coil.

I had just spent six years with Rami, a Middle Eastern businessman, with whom I shared in life little more than our mutual reverie about the life we wanted to share. He would take my hands in his and say, "You don't have to work. You don't need to worry about anything. I will take care of your student loans, everything. We will travel at will, you can write or whatever makes you happy."

I would be manic with ideas, practically panting at the ornament of my dream life dangled before me. Yes, we would travel to Egypt and Lebanon. I could smell the Arabian jasmine and apple hookah. I wanted an exotic life and one that was easy and creative. But I knew by now how this would play out. There would be a brief period of euphoria, drunk on a cocktail of our own imaginations, and we would wake up a few months later, hung over and staring at each other flatly over pasta in some restaurant. I knew, at some point, that he would never follow through with his promises, but I kept coming back for more. What was I looking for?

I wanted to be rescued, too. I had crippling student loan debt and Manhattan rent. And who wouldn't want a glamorous life? Adventure had always appealed to me more than any other quality a man had to offer. But my disappointment had taught me that if I wanted an extraordinary life, I had to be extraordinary myself. Whatever he promised, I would give it to myself. I decided to travel to the Middle East. On my own.

Cassie booked a two-hour session for our next meeting. She was notably deflated, without the typical incongruent exclamation marks at the ends of her sentences. She began, as usual, with a story, a monolithic wall of breathless words.

"It was a Thursday morning, two days before we we're supposed to leave for New Orleans. I pulled into the parking lot of a drugstore to get some travel supplies, and I saw Cole walking out of a breakfast café, walking arm in arm with a woman. I literally froze for a moment, then

I turned around and got back in my car. I decided to follow them and realized as I was following him that he was driving a different car. He drove me to the lake house in a Mercedes, and he was driving her in a Toyota Corolla. He pulled into the parking lot of an apartment complex and parked. They got out and they stood by the car and kissed and then she got in a car and drove away. He began walking toward an apartment when I jumped out of my car and ran up to catch him at his door. He was in shock. I told him that I saw everything. He asked me to come inside. He explained calmly that, yes, he is dating that woman because that's what you do when you're online dating—one dates multiple people—and that he was sorry that I had to see it. He said that it didn't change that he was excited about me and that he was excited about New Orleans."

She didn't seem to acknowledge his point and continued to relay the details of the incident.

"So, I said, 'Cole, I thought you lived downtown in a condo? And where is the Mercedes? I'm confused.'"

He said, "You would be worried about that. I was right about you. Look, I rented the car for our date and the lake house belongs to my uncle."

"You fucking asshole!"

"Really? Maybe I just know what women want. They want the fancy car and two houses. If I want to get a woman's attention, that's what I have to do. I'm just playing the game."

"You just want to get laid!"

"True. And that's your price."

"I'm not a prostitute!"

"Well, if all women want is evidence that you have money, then why should I want anything more than sex from you?"

"I thought we really shared something special at the lake house. I'm such an idiot!"

"No, you're not, we did. I was going to take you to New Orleans with my own money and I was going to tell you the truth because I really do like you."

The Women on My Couch

Despite their pretenses, both secretly yearned for a real relationship. Cole told Cassie that he wanted to keep dating her. He'd already bought their tickets to New Orleans and she had to decide if she was going to go.

"I don't get it. All these guys I meet online are just trying to hook up with as many women as possible. They're just out for sex. I feel used."

She began to sob. There would be no Knight in Shining Armor. Just when she thought she was special, another woman emerged victorious—again. I welled up right along with her. All I could do was sit and demonstrate that someone cared to see her pain.

She took a deep breath and began to collect.

"I don't know if I should go to New Orleans. I'm still attracted to him. But after getting the truth out of him, I now know that he has an MBA, and he's trying to start his own business, which is not currently solvent. He's an upstart. His apartment had one old couch, a card table for a kitchen table, no art."

I explored Cassie's capacity to accept a man for his truth. Most of what I'd heard were expectations—ideas about what men *should* be—all accepted, reinforced even, by her mother, sisters, and friends. But when stated as a declaration of rights, her demands would look something like this:

A man should make a good living: enough to buy a condo and a lake house—yet have ample time to pay attention to you. He should want to relieve you of all of your burdens, debt, hard work so that you can relax at home with children—then when he walks in the door, he should spontaneously desire to throw you against a wall and tear your clothes off. He must demonstrate competence in the following areas: driving, handy work, oral sex, and other various feats of masculinity. The ability to chop logs is a bonus. He should buy you a Chanel handbag as a gesture of love, enjoy shopping for new bath towels, wipe your nose when you're sick, hold you when you're upset (without trying to tell you what to do), spank you like Christian Grey and then read you a Rumi poem right after, all of this without you having to ask, of course.

I know this is hyperbole, but there is truth in these expectations. Are they attainable or even sustainable in a relationship? When guys don't live up, women can get turned off—even outraged and contemptuous that men aren't exactly who we think they should be: Brad Pitt.

When you look into the living room and all you see is some dude in his boxers playing video games, it's a powerful moment of truth. The reality is that some men are depressed, incompetent, or anxious, ingratiating pleasers. A bunch of them have no skills for seduction. Some wear holey socks, forget your birthday, and don't help with the laundry. Some make less money than you.

Sure, none of this is sexy. Fine.

But as one of my girlfriends said to me, "When I don't know how to use the remote control and he has to show me how for the fifth time, he doesn't get fundamentally turned off by me."

It's fine for women to *want* men to provide, protect, thrill, or even save them, but this extends beyond wanting. When a want goes unfulfilled, we feel disappointed. The rancor that builds inside women when men aren't Prince Charming suggests that these aren't just preferences, they're demands.

These unrealistic expectations destroy libido and ruin relationships. Obliging men to be our saviors is really just dependency disguised. It takes a strong woman to allow a man to be a human being. A woman who can confront her own fears. I had to remind myself these things— even as the words came out of my mouth. We all have a deep yearning for safety, to be taken care of by some omnipotent being.

"Cassie, there is no Prince Charming."

She sat silent.

"Can you take Cole as he is?"

"No."

She decided not to go to New Orleans, and it probably was a wise decision. Even though she was disappointed, she recovered quickly. But the larger lesson, about who she was and who she wanted a man to be, was now being reevaluated—and this, certainly, would bring her closer to finding the love she was looking for.

The Women on My Couch

I hate to be the Cinderella slayer. In therapy, the first step toward growth is grieving the loss of the Prince Charming fantasy. From there, a new sense of confidence begins. Cassie had to learn to armor up, strap on the sword, and mount the horse.

Lilu

Of all my clients, one truly ruffled me. She was more secure, more certain. A psychologist generally prefers to be in control. We diagnose, challenge, devise treatment plans, and direct the questions. The psychologist is an expert, possessing a skill set for change or relief. The client hopes, but doesn't know when or how exactly, this relief will come. But Lilu took the reins in our first session, leaving me to sit with the uncertainty—perhaps as it should be.

Lilu made a compelling argument against love. She had many lovers, often at the same time.

"I won't keep a man around for any longer than a year," she declared.

"Part-timers," she called them, "are more efficient than one full-timer. I get more attention this way." Moreover, Lilu instructed, "*My* attention is limited, so they have to fight for it."

"Do they know about each other?"

"Oh yeah. Keeps them on their toes. I am not a woman who gets taken for granted."

I simply followed her lead. I was having a hard time finding a problem with this setup. Any feelings she had for these guys were shallow and fleeting. *Love is missing*, I thought, she must want love.

"Don't you want to fall in love?" I asked.

"No," she answered without hesitation. "I do get some romantic feelings, but nothing to be sad over if lost."

How could she not want love? I felt a bit defensive, ready to find some diagnosis for this aberrant woman who defied the holiest of virtues. But I also felt a strange admiration. She was living the ultimate wish fulfillment, a female sultan with her own harem of men competing for her affections, a life that I could never have because I was about to get married. I had signed the dotted line for love. I would listen to Lilu and wonder if her lifestyle was a superior choice. Entertaining this fantasy put my happiness in question. So, I doubled down on her.

"Do you want a deeper connection with someone?" I pressed.

She squinted at me.

"What for?" she asked.

I wasn't sure where to go next. Lilu really had her dating situation under tight control. She seemed the antithesis of the dependent types who put all of their eggs in one basket. She had lots of baskets. Her needs were met, and this made my job hard. Attention, approval, power; if a client isn't aching for anything, she is usually disinclined to change.

This was how Lilu wanted to begin therapy, to lead not with her problem but with the exultation of her lifestyle. Once in a while, people come to therapy and proceed to tell the therapist that they know everything: the problem, the solution, and all sundry answers to life. She was like sitting with a rebellious teenager or an alcoholic in denial. I feel the urge to remind such people that *I'm not the principal* or *I'm not your fill-in-the-blank parent*. I want to say, *I'm cool, you can tell me anything*. But it doesn't matter what I think I am. What matters is who *they* think I am.

Lilu was in her mid-twenties and she spoke with efficiency and certitude, as if she didn't have time to fritter away on mawkish stories of her past. She lived in trendy Echo Park, home of artist collectives, vintage clothiers, fabricators of hand-stitched leather bags made on site—lots of little hipster hobbits busily crafting their wares. Lilu had a bigger vision than this scene. Ivy-League-educated and with a degree in art history, she never found a job, so she decided to start an Internet venue for artisanal fashion. She was a first-generation immigrant from South Africa who pleased her parents with academic achievement but decided to follow her dream to be in fashion against her parents' wishes. She had organized a group of young designers to sell through her venue. The only hitch was that she had outrageous student loan debt from her private school education and not a lot of capital for her business—but she had a strategy for that problem.

"I'm on a website called Seeking Arrangement. A sugar daddy situation. He provides you a monthly allowance, and you become his friend. I have two men, both in their fifties, who each give me $5,000 a month. I put all of it into the business. Both men think I'm some subservient immigrant—a fetish which I find offensive—but might as well play that role and benefit from their ignorance. They just want to be served and cared for—I get that people need that."

"What's it like for you to go on dates with them?"

"I see each of them once a week. It's not bad at all. I enjoy their company and I try to make them feel what they want to feel—sexual, alive. They want fun. They want the simple things that get lost in life. It makes me happy to provide that for them."

"How's the sex?"

"Transactional sex can be hot. Or being told what to do by an older man can be hot. And since they're paying me so much, I know I have to work to keep them interested, so that keeps me sharp."

Lilu was satisfied on all levels: financial, sexual, and emotional. This wasn't the tale of a disadvantaged woman reduced to sex work. I was intrigued. High-pay arrangements are glamorous in the fantasy minds of many women. She certainly didn't struggle with low libido like the masses of monogamous women who more often graced my couch. She enjoyed men, but her life wasn't consumed by the pursuit of love. She told me that she had her priorities in proper order:

"I think about hiring software engineers and factories in Mexico and finding up-and-coming fashion designers. I read the *Wall Street Journal*, not *Cosmo*. I have a broader vision for my life."

I considered her perspective. She was a modern woman exercising her choice, and she was very conscious about creating an alternative lifestyle. How many of us date with the end goal of marriage? There was something to be said for the bravery it took to follow an unconventional path. I was even a tad jealous. She likely made more money than I. Was I on the wrong end of the sex industry? My therapeutic neutrality was all askew, and I vacillated back to suspicion. This couldn't be the new halcyon way. She was, in fact, in the office of a therapist. *So, is this really what liberation looks like?* I wondered.

California has always been a beacon for seekers of self-determination. Midwestern artistic hopefuls, immigrants, gangsters, New Age spiritual questers all hustle, fight, and forge. This town may brim with creative energy, health, and beauty, but it is not a happy place. The dark side of the struggle to succeed is being self-centered. Ambitions come first, relationships last. Loneliness is one of the top complaints in my office. And, unlike other feelings, loneliness doesn't pass. The social fabric of L.A. is transient. Few people have a steady paycheck, and self-images flutter according to the whims of script readers or casting agents. Then there is the narcissistic injury of those who wanted to overcome child-hood rejection by becoming famous—only to be rejected over and over again.

Lilu was confident, but I wondered if she was happy. At the end of the first session, she revealed why she was in my office. She had suddenly lost her ability to have an orgasm. When a full-functioning woman abruptly loses her orgasm, something is going on. There is a mystery to unravel.

"Is this happening with all of your lovers or just one?"

"Just one. The Professor."

"What is sex like with him?"

"He's boring in bed. Very vanilla. He recently said 'I love you' and I was like, 'Oh, God, he's trying to make love to me.' He wants attention and he disrupts me from my fantasy and then I can't get off," she said, rolling her eyes with contempt.

Lilu had been dating The Professor, casually of course, for a few months. The only times she smiled was while describing him, until she recalled a fight they had at a recent dinner. Over conversation about current events, she became adversarial. "I kept disagreeing with him, and he was getting annoyed, but I couldn't stop. It wasn't about the is-sue. I don't actually care about warring factions in Syria. I was getting some bizarre pleasure at creating this rancor between us. At the end of the evening, we would normally go back to his place, but he said he was tired and wanted to go home alone."

She was insightful enough to notice an unexplained impulse to create animosity. I wondered what she felt threatened by. If not his knowledge of world events, then what really triggered her to attack?

"Let's go back to the memory of your dinner date. Can you remember what you felt before talking about Syria?"

"Hmm. A fondness for him. I think I respect him more than the other guys I've dated. I'm impressed by him."

"How do you feel about yourself around him?"

"Suddenly aware of how much I don't know, so I feel slightly off balance, not as sure of myself. I'm used to feeling grounded in my intelligence. My whole identity is built around being the smart girl."

I appreciated that she was allowing a moment of vulnerability. But I jumped on it too quickly.

"Perhaps your jabs at him were an attempt to reestablish your sense of worth."

She diverted the conversation by launching into a series of stories about the other guys she was dating, all which seemed totally irrelevant. She talked very fast, and when I tried to speak, she actually lifted her hand to halt me. I sat back in my chair and listened for a theme; it was all about her bravado with men, what a great lover she was.

Supercilious clients don't like the therapist to make interpretations. They have to make the connections. It's a delicate balance. On the basis of my experience, I knew that I had to ask questions and follow her or she'd turn against me. Instead of challenging her, I aligned with her defense.

"That's great, that you're enjoying yourself. You want me to know that, that your lifestyle is great."

She set down her bottle of kombucha and began gesticulating in that careful manner one does when comfortable, even pleased, to be in one's own skin.

"Right, I think porn is the problem. I think I've watched so much I'm dependent on it. Now I can't get off without it."

"Any preferences in your porn viewing?" I always ask this question, because sometimes the content people are drawn to is psychologically revelatory.

"Amateur stuff is best. The professionals all seem like they're trying too hard, they're so overwrought it's funny."

"Any particular acts that you like watching?"

"I like to watch women dommes. Men-as-slave or –houseboy scenarios."

I tend to examine my client's emotional relationship to pornography to understand why a compulsion develops. Porn can serve psychological functions beyond the simple titillations of the body. Her preferences were consistent with her love of power, not an area of deficit. I wasn't sold porn was the actual problem in her orgasm situation.

"Do you act this out with The Professor?"

"No, I haven't shared my tastes with him, which is unusual. Maybe because I like him. My mind doesn't want to put him in that kind of role."

"Tell me what you like about him."

She smiled broadly.

"You smiled!"

I liked her. She was candid and fearless and I enjoyed listening to the way she had it all figured out.

"Can we talk about it, liking this guy more than usual?"

"I hate feeling mushy about a guy. It's a loss of composure. Control, maybe?"

Fighting can be an effective way to create distance. The act of asserting strong opinions helped Lilu remember her identity and recover a sense of control—not over him, but over her own feelings. This girl did not want to want. Sex was strength, desire weakness.

In the bedroom, while the dependent types neurotically attach love to sex, the withdrawal types neurotically *detach* love from sex. I wondered if Lilu was acting out a pattern of avoidance. All day I hear stories of people who need some measure of distance in order to handle other people. Some can't look into each other's eyes, or they require role-play, or they can orgasm only from some facing-away position like doggy style. Women are often characterized as requiring emotional closeness to be sexual, but for women like Lilu, the opposite is true. She rejected love and had developed an entire belief system that supported her aversion.

"Having enough distance is important to you," I said, hoping she'd see that her pride was her defense mechanism.

"Independence. I like my freedom, and when men get too close, it ruins everything. I don't want my life taken over by a relationship. I want to puke when I see billboards for Nicholas Sparks's movies. Naïve romantics are the new Victorians—the pursuit of love itself is oppressive. All of your creative energies are put into the pursuit and maintenance of romance. You know that quote by Louisa May Alcott, 'Liberty is a better husband than love'—that is my motto."

Her cell phone alarm went off. Rather than waiting for me to cue the end of a session, she made sure she never took more than the allotted 45 minutes. She began to gather her bag as I made a final comment.

"It seems like your body is sensitive to any threat to your sense of independence. You can't relax into an orgasm, so something far deeper is at work in you. Your body is really responding to something here."

When we're not conscious of our fears, the vagina lets us know. The body speaks a subtle language. A vague impulse to recoil, a sudden fatigue or blankness in the bedroom, and irritation for no reason are whispers from the unconscious. When she gets too close, an internal sensor is triggered, and she instinctively retreats. Some women shut down by spending more time away from home, by taking more time to be alone, or even by starting a fight. Flirting and affection might be avoided. It's a protective mechanism, a sign of a togetherness tension.

Lilu got under my skin. I'd think of her words as I fell asleep at night or when I took a shower. Her certainty triggered me, as if she were more grounded than I was. In my own life, I was approaching unfamiliar territory. I was about to move in with my husband after having lived most of my adult life with roommates. My relationship style was always on the autonomous end of the spectrum. I'd never rejected love, but I'd always been a space- and freedom-loving, marriage-doubting woman. I felt, acutely, the vulnerability in dedicating myself to one man. As I explored Lilu's point of view, I was also thinking of my own decisions. A part of me had always wanted to be like her. Lilu saw herself as the actualization of The Liberated Woman—but I was beginning to think she was confusing emotional with political liberation.

The visage of a liberated woman has evolved throughout American history. When it comes to defining what this term means today, the process is very individualized and vague. An overlooked time when the issue of liberation was more clear and burning was the flapper rebellion of the 1920s. This period saw the great dismantling of every aspect of traditional womanhood. Emancipating their bodies in the most literal way, flappers were the first to shed the corsets and long, heavy skirts. They took up sports for the first time and—even more vulgar—they danced the Charleston. It was the Jazz Age and women were showing up at nightclubs, getting drunk, and smoking cigarettes. They hit on men. They took lovers. Many lovers. Even lesbianism was in vogue.

It was post–World War I, and the scope of loss, the collective trauma, and the unraveling of society sent some people into party mode. Much to the mortification of their parents, flappers were a bunch of hedonistic hellcats bent on not returning to the way life had been—ever. For these subversive ladies, liberation was about defiance. They weren't just early lushes; they were trailblazers. Their mothers were confined to domesticity. Flappers worked and they traveled; they bought cars. Their mothers wore their hair long, piled in loose buns, and no makeup. The "flaming youth," as the media referred to them, cut their hair into short bobs and wore red lipstick and smoky eyeliner. Eschewing the image of women's gentility, they tried on tough attitudes and swearing, saying words like "horsefeathers" (and "darn"). These ladies led a sexual revolution that unfortunately was short lived. The Great Depression hit, and we reverted to conservativism and remained there until the next revolution.

As the flappers carved out new social freedoms, they, like us, had to balance their objectives against their emotional desires. They had broken out and then had to confront new questions: How to balance sexual freedom with love? Self-determination with marriage or children? This idea of independence carries the notion that freedom means unlimited possibility. Relationships, however, introduce limits. Our biological clock introduces limits. Way before our "Can she have it all—career *and* family" question, these ladies navigated the edges of their limits.

Most of the famous flappers chose to love. And the modern-day single folks who sit in my office, they continue to desire romance all the same. Every once in a while I get a client who repudiates love altogether. None had been as strident as Lilu. I took her point of view seriously. Could rejecting love be a form of independence? Was Lilu a contemporary trailblazer, hacking out a new frontier beyond the confines of the emotional limits of commitment, loyalty, and monogamy?

Lilu's reaction to intimacy and her need for autonomy around men were so strong, I knew there had to be a personal history. To fully understand an erotic psyche, it's actually important to consider a person's relationship with her parents. Often, my clients don't initially see why I need to ask about their mother or father if they're just coming in to talk about orgasms. But erotic tastes are rooted in our histories, and erotic maps are drawn from unique life experiences.

I learned from Lilu that her mother was overbearing, focusing constant attention on Lilu's academic development and extracurricular activities, such as playing the violin and running track. Lilu felt like her mother's little trophy child. Little attention was placed on Lilu's actual emotional experience. There was very little affection in this family, a family held together by commitment, loyalty, and shared values—all of which Lilu began to distrust as empty ties that forced her into compliance. Lilu internalized her parents' ideals, excelling at school, performing in national competitions, and shutting down her needs for affection, focusing instead on perfection. She decided that desiring affection was weak, that successful people were focused and strong, above such trifling soppiness. I didn't know if I could help her uncover a need for love, but maybe The Professor would. If she didn't sabotage it first.

"Don't you want to experience desire for someone?" I asked.

"I have and I hated it." She fixed her kohl-rimmed eyes on mine. "My first boyfriend cheated on me. I was eighteen. The most painful realization was that even the closest person in your life has the potential to lie, to leave, or to simply change his mind and choose another woman. That's what happened. He decided he was into somebody else. The capriciousness of that struck me more than the betrayal. You know, I wasn't morally outraged, I was more disturbed by the truth of human nature."

She spoke in a jaded, tough tone that was very cool, superior even, but I could feel a flicker of her sadness.

"You discovered there is no way to control love."

"Attraction can't be controlled, so why make myself helpless to it? I had the nicest, most decent guy. He wasn't a liar. He told me about her. He was a good guy and we were really close—yet still there was no guarantee of safety. So, I swore that I would never love only one man again."

"So, now you're safe."

She nodded. I was glad she was sharing more of her story, but I noted that no emotion registered on her face as she spoke about such a formative moment in her life, one with enough impact to drive an entire lifestyle.

Finally, Lilu's rigid defense of her philosophical disdain for love was making sense psychologically. Even though Lilu had a "never again" mentality, she didn't want to be alone. With all of her lovers, each in a neat little compartment, she was able to both connect and withdraw. She fought a constant internal battle: the need to be loved versus the fear of intimacy. Instead of loving, she made people love her.

"You like this guy, but then there is a moment when you want to pull away. Can we zero in on what you felt that moment before you felt suffocated?"

"Exposed somehow, that I like him and am totally open to him, body and heart."

"Yes, having an orgasm, is a surrender. There is a letting go—a moment of being out of control—especially in the presence of a man you actually like. Perhaps, there is something symbolic about that?"

Lilu was too acutely vulnerable to have an orgasm. If they can handle it, vulnerability helps people access passion. But the anxiety had exceeded Lilu's window of tolerance. If she wasn't open hearted, she wasn't going to feel much. Lilu had exchanged passion for the ego aggrandizement of adoration, which ostensibly had its own euphoria.

But passion was my agenda. Lilu valued safety over ecstasy, and she took pride in being an "independent woman." I was beginning to view her posture as a pseudo-independence driven by panic, a classic defense used when people experience a sense of shame about needing other people. Independence isn't about isolation; it's about holding on to yourself in the presence of others.

Lilu's approach to relating was utilitarian. Pragmatic and transactional at times, yet still sufficiently erotic for her tastes. And she was right, there was no avoiding hurt in committed relationships. She viewed loyalty or commitment as unnecessary in the modern world. With the sheer numbers of available single people on the market, it wasn't necessary to make the painful compromises required by loyalty. Loyalty was really just fear disguised as principle. I headed home, always energized from a bandy about with Lilu—part afraid and part gratified that my life was now different.

I was the first to move in. I would have our new apartment to myself for one week. Standing in the empty 1920s Spanish bungalow, the sun shining in on the blank white walls and starkly clean kitchen, I realized I had in front of me a blank slate. About to build something that wasn't just for me, each end table, lamp, and popcorn maker seemed suddenly precious. There was none of the anxiety I had anticipated, none of the old skepticisms about cohabitation. Only exuberance. I painted the walls bright pink and turquoise and purple.

The Women on My Couch

As I painted, I thought about how Lilu spent a great deal of time with men for someone who placed so little value on them. I remembered her words, and she started to sound less convincing to me:

"I know you think I have a control problem, but I'm not going to sacrifice my happiness to some guy with whims I can't change—and I'm fortunate that I don't have to. This isn't really about morals, it's about practicality. We don't need to tether ourselves to one person and feel sanctimonious about it. We can float freely in and out of people's lives. I'm not concerned about infidelity, not biting my nails when a guy doesn't text, and I don't deal with guys who've lost interest and would rather read Reddit than talk to me or who prefer to get it on with double-D blondes in tacky outfits acting like little girls and all manner of dopes like that. Don't have to deal. This is peace."

Something was missing from her hyper-sovereign utopia. I wasn't so enamored by her anymore. I began to experience a sensation around Lilu that was similar to the one I had while researching the stories of famous flappers. Originally, looking for inspiration, I'd read books and diaries, and then grew tired of their saccharine stories of love affair after love affair. It was like staying at the party too long. Many seemed self-involved to a pukey excess. Definitely not my Aphrodite's.

All revolutions have their figureheads, people who represent the ideal, whom others want to follow. For the flaming youth generation, it was Clara Bow, a movie star who often played the quintessential flapper. She inspired throngs of young women across the country. Clara Bow's roles came to define what it meant to be a modern woman. Clara was widely known as the It Girl—a euphemism for the still unspeakable, unsavory phrase "sex appeal." She appeared in a movie called *It* (1927) that made this word part of the popular lexicon and Clara Bow an icon.

I watched the movie *It*, and Clara's charm still resonated. It's a black-and-white silent film that begins with the definition of "it" printed on the screen, as defined by the writer and producer, Elinor Glyn:

> IT is that quality possessed by some which draws all others by magnetic force. With IT you can win all men if you are a

woman—and all women if you are a man. It can be a quality of the mind as well as physical attraction. The possessor of IT must be entirely unself-conscious. Self-confidence and indifference as to whether you are pleasing or not.

Clara Bow plays a vivacious shop girl, with smoky doe eyes and a broad red smile, from a working-class neighborhood. She has "it." Basically, she seduces a hot CEO who already had a fancy girlfriend, a stuffy blonde socialite who dons the bob and makeup but who holds on to the stolid Old World manners, which is a bore. The theme of this movie is overt—it literally seeks to define sex appeal. Clara flouts traditional mores and helps release women from the obligation to please mothers, husbands, neighbors, and ministers. Liberation in this period was akin to a female insurgency, but there was major backlash.

Despite their social influence, not everybody approved. In 1926, the House of Representatives literally had a debate about skirt length. Chicago police had a unit to protect public morals and would bother women swimming at Lake Michigan to measure the distance between bathing suit and knee. Violators of skirt length were put in the back of a paddy wagon and hauled to the police station. A book came out called *Fascinating Womanhood*, akin to a vintage version of *The Rules.* A woman was advised to seduce a man by presenting as weak, innocent, and child-like.

Flappers didn't care.

But they also, famously, didn't care about much beyond themselves. Flappers were not into politics, voting rights, or labor activism. In a similar way, Lilu had this privilege of hard-won rights, and yet, there was no sense of ethics, justice, or honor in her freedom. Perhaps there is more to being cool than a rebellious attitude.

Do we have some responsibility that goes along with our independence? We can love as we want, but should we have ethics? This has been a question on my mind as I'm confronted daily in my private practice with the dark side of human sexuality: selfishness, sadism, exploitation, sex addiction. I'm not interested in moralizing—not that morals or values have to be oppressive—but being a therapist and being married, I've learned how to care for others more deeply. My husband once said to me, "If you hurt me, you hurt yourself." I realized that I was part of a system and that I had an impact, whether I liked it or not. We all are. Single or married.

Being married has inspired me to be better than I once was. When I look into his eyes and see the precious vulnerability of a man who gave me his heart, I see no small token. This offering I want to hold dear. When I sit with clients each day, both the predators and the prey, I can't help but think that our little decisions in love have ripple effects across a larger system of interaction.

To me other notable women of the flapper era who were equally bold were more inspiring than the flappers. Women like Carrie Chapman Catt, founder of the League of Women Voters and leader of the Voting Rights movement. And Jane Edna Hunter, an African American woman who started a shelter for black women seeking refuge in the North that eventually became the Working Girls Association, a vaunted vocational training center, and she herself obtained a law degree. Margaret Sanger, founder of Planned Parenthood. And there was Eleanor Roosevelt, who encouraged women to run for office and to use their newly acquired voting rights to vote each other into all levels of government.

Lilu had conflated independence with individualism. Interdependence was confused with dependence, which is associated with loss: loss of dreams, loss of hard-won freedom, and loss of self.

The final crack in Lilu's façade came with the revelation of one missing detail. She was faking orgasms. She could've told The Professor that she wasn't having orgasms, but she chose to actively lie. She even hid this fact from me. Yes, faking orgasms is common, and we do if for many reasons: to make him feel good about himself or perhaps to make him stop or to help him have an orgasm. It's quite pragmatic. But the inauthenticity of a dramatic show of sounds and movement is striking to me. If Lilu was truly independent emotionally, then why not be real?

I took a few weeks off and traveled to the Dominican Republic. I sat down for a beer in Santo Domingo with Dr. Rafael Garcia, a sex

researcher and professor, to discuss our work with women's sexual issues. I was curious about the similarities and differences in sexual behavior in the United States and the Caribbean. My first question was,
"Are Dominican women as gloriously sexual as Americans imagine
them to be?" hoping his answer would be yes. He smiled broadly and
said, "No. In fact, many are shy and inhibited. The most common issue
I see if low libido."

"Noooo! But the Bachata dancing and the miniskirts?"

"They're struggling with the religious repression of Catholicism and
a high rate of sexual abuse."

"Why do we think that?" I wondered aloud.

"Myth, projection—and lots of faking." He told me that there is a
high incidence of faking orgasms, just as there is in the United States.

I'd thought about how women are good at separating behavior from
desire. We're guilty of being seductive and sexy and sexual—without
the faintest feelings of lust. Dr. Garcia told me that the Dominican
Republic has a "prostitution-accepting culture" and that the motivation for sex is often associated with nonsexual factors: money, security,
approval.

This chasm between truth and action must have consequences for the
psyche. Most women in the United States don't fake orgasms because
their economic survival is on the line; we more often do it out of social
fear or desire for approval. What does that say about our independence
from men if we can't tell them we're not pleased?

Finding freedom in the context of a relationship is at the core of my
work with women of all ages. From the nineteen twenties to today,
autonomy has been an evolving process rather than an achieved state.
Because we don't exist in isolation, there will always be some guy, or
kids, or parents, or bigger forces in society that challenge our self-sov-
ereignty. In college, I'd tell my girlfriends that we should live together
for the rest of our lives in a big house full of women. Men could come
and go on the side. And, indeed, I lived most of my adult life in this very
arrangement, though it wasn't an intentional commune but more out

of economic necessity. Either way, I loved it. I loved keeping my daily affairs separate from my love affairs, the comradery, and the freedom. When my husband proposed, I didn't say no for a simple reason: I couldn't deny happiness. I knew I'd wrestle with feeling constricted living as a couple, so right away, I strived for a sense of balance. A space where freedom is not defined by cutting off from men. Nor is it defined by relationships. It's a balance of being in relationship to a man—and the world around you—while holding your own ground.

Lilu returned for a last time. I'd replaced my couch with a traditional Freudian-style chaise lounge. Almost all of my clients were perplexed by it. Nobody wanted to lie down. They'd rather sit on the edge with no back to lean against. But Lilu walked in, took off her heels, and reclined on my divan, one arm perched on the pillows, an iced coffee in the other hand.

"I broke it off with him. When it stops being fun, that's when I'm out. People never really change, so why not stop now and remember the good times."

"What do you feel?"

"I'll miss him, but I'm OK. I have the wisdom to know that it wasn't going to work."

Lilu never showed consideration for the impact her behavior had on the men in her life. I didn't want to push my ideals about love on her; she had a right to her own philosophy. But what is the social outcome when we interact only for its immediate practical value to us? When is exercising freedom really just an excuse for anomie? What if we all rejected vulnerability, commitment, and loyalty? I wondered if it was fair for me to even ask such questions of women given our history of sexual regulation. Society may not ask these questions of men, but I do. As men and women take turns sitting on my couch all day, each lamenting the dating world from their own point of view, that juxtaposition brings into sharp relief the cycle of injuries that become belief systems and then behaviors and, finally, large-scale patterns and generalizations.

Lilu was talking, and I faded out, noticing her bridled shoulders back, head high, distancing from me.

"Seems like you don't need much from me."

"Yeah, I think I've eliminated the issue."

Lilu did not change as a result of our brief time together. Rather, I was the one who had shifted. Because her beliefs tapped into a long standing ambivalence of my own, I'd thought about what I wanted moving forward and decided that, in marriage, I'd relinquish selfishness, not freedom. Well, in theory at least.

The Professor tried to get Lilu back, texting, calling, showing up at her apartment, to no avail. She likely provoked feelings of neediness in him—probably an outward expression of Lilu's split off desires.

I'd sat once, alone on my chair before a session, and tried to conjure compassion for Lilu, but it's hard to feel for a client who won't feel. I thought of her childhood, that once she must have longed to be loved. I sensed that deep down she was angry, sadistic. When I'm able to access that anger in clients like Lilu, the real hurt is right there, underneath, and therapy has a shot at being effective.

Lilu didn't stick around with me to address her anger. She wasn't the type to have an ongoing relationship with a therapist; she certainly wasn't going to *need* me. Ideally, she would have stayed with me and eventually would have wanted from me, and I would have given to her in hopes of creating what clinicians call the "corrective emotional experience," where we provide love, a stable love that changes what the client expects from the world. But in reality clients like Lilu won't let me get that close. She terminated therapy by simply not showing up for her last scheduled appointment. No good-bye, no thank you. I was hurt. I really did enjoy her and wished to be a transformative presence in her life.

In what had turned out to be our last session, I tried one more time. I had said to Lilu, "I acknowledge that you're enjoying your lifestyle, but it depends on a constant external source—"

"There are a lot of men in Los Angeles," she interjected.

Melissa

An empty plate, save for a few uneaten brussels sprouts, sat in the middle of the living room floor. The remains of a romantic evening, now covered in furry white patches; a sulfurous odor wafted through the cozy room of couches, books, and picture frames. The little decomposed balls of cruciferous vegetables sat silently, yet their presence was a clarion call about love, marriage, and equality.

Melissa and Garrett had been married only six months. Excited to nest, each night she'd come home from work and cook dinner. She was ceremonious about it, too, opening bottles of wine, arranging little French cheese plates, setting the table with candles. This wasn't typical for her—just high spirits about sharing a home with the man she loved. Melissa began to notice that he rarely offered to do the dishes. And further, he often left his plate in the place where he'd eaten—on the table, on the couch, on the floor. She tried to make sense of this incongruous behavior mottling her blissful evenings. *Wasn't there a social rule that if someone cooks, the other cleans? Does he expect me to cook, clear, and wash? That would be chauvinist. My husband isn't a chauvinist.*

So, Melissa set up a test. One night, after finishing a dish of pork chops stuffed with smoked Gouda and a side of brussels sprouts, he set his plate on the floor and invited her over to the couch to make love. Afterward, Melissa left his dish exactly where he'd put it—on the living room floor.

Five days passed.

She said nothing. He said nothing. They sat on the couch watching TV, walked past the rotting food hundreds of times to reach the front door—all while the little sprouts just sat there—as a struggle over how to share a life eddied in the air.

Melissa could still remember speaking her marriage vows. She'd recited the traditional promises to love, honor, and cherish. Each word rolling slowly from her tongue as she allowed herself to register the meaning of *honor, cherish*, with full reverence for their gravity. She was full of pride and eager devotion; the vows were an initiation into a family and a community, a deeply spiritual moment.

Nobody told her that marriage was actually a constant inconvenience. Everything about merging two lives felt hard. She wanted to spend Saturdays trawling farmers markets and hiking. He wanted to golf with his friends and watch football. He wanted sex in the morning. She wanted coffee. Even the way they went to the store together was discordant. She brought a list and coupons. He randomly picked up whatever he fancied, running through the store haphazardly as she went from one aisle to the next, carefully considering the meals she was planning. He was happy to eat cereal and sandwiches three times a day. All the small things that everyone tells you don't matter, you know, as long as you have love, were making her want to harm him in his sleep.

Melissa came to me after the brussels sprouts incident because their housekeeper, who came once a week, was the one to pick up the plate. Melissa sat in my waiting room, her eyes cast downward and the corner of her lip trembling. She walked into my office, and tears were falling before she could speak. She looked like a reserved woman who'd been moved beyond her limits of propriety. I like when clients show up in a raw state. There's no resistance, no hidden truth to dig for. It's all at the surface, exposed. I sat her down on my couch.

"Tell me what the tears are about."

"I made a mistake in choosing a husband. But what can I do? My parents paid so much money for the wedding, if I divorce him, I would look disrespectful and frivolous," she said, exhaling as if defeated. A wisp of blonde hair fell across her eyes, and she didn't bother to move it.

"Sorry I'm crying."

I handed her a tissue.

"You seem to be reacting as though you're grieving a loss—like there's no hope left."

She sat silent, shoulders slumped, and then reanimated with a hostile tone.

"I never thought I'd fall into this cliché situation. How did I let this happen to me? We both work the same amount of hours, yet I am the one who stops to buy groceries or folds laundry. I've tried to tell him what I expect and he acts so annoyed, like I'm his nagging mother. I'm trapped. Fuck! Sorry. Sorry, I said 'fuck.' "

I set up a chair in front of Melissa and asked her to pretend Garrett was sitting there. She stood up and looked at the chair for a moment. Where there is anger, there is still hope.

"Be as irrational as you want. Tell him how angry you are—and you can say fuck as many times as you want," I instructed.

She was initially hesitant, and then she fixed her gaze on the chair.

"What the fuck is wrong with you? Are you a child? Didn't anybody teach you manners?"

She started to cry.

"Don't give up. Stay with your anger."

She took a breath and straightened her posture.

"Do you think I'm your servant? Do you think a woman is supposed to take care of you? Do you think I want to look at your shit all over the place? I live here, too. Have some damn respect."

"Time to switch. Act *him* out for me," I directed.

She slouched down on the couch and in a mocking voice, "I do a lot for this house. I take out the trash. I walk the dog. I feed the dog. You don't even appreciate what I do. When I get home from work, I want to relax. I'd rather hang out with you than do work."

That didn't have the effect I wanted. "Now switch back to you," I directed.

"I want to hang out, too, but somebody has to do the work. It's part of life; stuff has to get done. If we do it together, it's over faster, and then we can both have fun."

She threw up her hands.

"This is where you get stuck?" I asked.

"Yes. I feel trapped, like we're both set in our point of view. This is why I stopped talking to him about it."

"Do you punish him?"

"Yes."

"Give that a voice." I wanted to pull all the rancor out to the surface so we could deal with it head-on.

"I'm on strike. No more sex. I'm not attracted to a little boy I have to take care of."

Melissa and Garrett were in a post marriage adjustment phase. When couples move in together, the differences come to the fore. All the little idiosyncrasies—how people manage time or organization or even sleep—are garishly exposed on a daily basis. Melissa's immediate reaction was to be judgmental. His way was wrong, hers was right. Her thoughts focused on how rude or lazy or imprudent he was, and she repeated them over and over in her head until she didn't see anything else in him but rude, lazy, imprudent.

Melissa showed no sign of understanding Garrett's point of view, and when I'd asked her to role-play him, she did so in a mocking voice. Sure, she was disappointed that he wasn't living up to her ideals, and at face value, her ideals didn't sound outrageous. They sounded like wishes for an egalitarian marriage. It was tempting to agree with her, and I caught myself thinking, *What a lout.* My clients bewail these Peter Pan boyfriends all the time—dudes who let the house turn into a junkyard while they play video games. And at this point in history, it seems like common sense that helping out around the house makes for a happier relationship. But no, many guys still don't get it, thinking she's just fussy. In therapy, I let these guys know what a colossal mistake they're making.

This dereliction of household duty taps into the collective outrage women have from the years of being stuck in servitude, which has led to a collective narrative with the wife cast as righteous victim and the husband (an often unwitting) villain. I didn't want to fall into the trap of reflexive judgment. I knew from doing couples therapy that her point of view was likely skewed and that underneath her equality expecta-tion was actually a demand—that the house (and the relationship) be maintained her way. This is not egalitarian. There was no respect for difference in lifestyle, no negotiation, and, as evidenced by the brussels sprouts incident, no communication. Melissa was a righteous victim, and Garrett was clearly a villain.

I sat alone at my desk late one evening after Melissa, my last client, had gone home. I pawed through my collection of vintage psychology books. The classics: Freud, Rogers, May, Horney all had the best writ-ing. They possessed a combination of poetic prose and sophisticated insights instead of facile advice. I knew exactly whose work would apply to Melissa's dilemma. I pulled a book from my shelf. The late psychiatrist and pioneer sex researcher Helen Singer Kaplan had an answer to why we fall into this perceptual snare. Sure, there is truth in Melissa's complaints, but Melissa seemed to have lost the broader picture of who Garrett was. Dr. Kaplan observed that women regulate their attraction downward, by a slow and steady narration of complaints about why he hasn't been an ideal partner: *he gets lost when he drives, he's a bad tipper, his socks smell.*

Melissa had been rehearsing these recriminations for months. But Kaplan says that this process can also happen in the opposite direc-tion, that we can turn ourselves on by switching to a positive gaze. The brain has a remarkable ability to sexualize just about anything or anyone. Kaplan says that humans are actually "distinguished by remark-able diversity, malleability and plasticity." With this ability, the brain can be conditioned to a variety of sexual stimuli. Women do not have a rigid and predetermined set of turn-ons. This is great news because it provides room for some control. We can use the power of the mind to our advantage.

I decided to try this with Melissa, to help her "up-regulate." If it didn't work, then we would be closer to the resistance, that internal force that blockades the change people want. It was evening and in preparation for our session, I lit some candles and plugged in my trickling fountain.

Melissa walked in, pert and jaunty, kale smoothie in hand. I asked her to lean back into the couch and put her feet up.

"Close your eyes and get a picture in your mind's eye of when you were first dating Garrett. Remember what was attractive about him."

"I'm thinking about his lips, his arms. I'm thinking about riding in his truck."

"Remember the way you anticipated a date or longed for him to touch you."

"OK, I can feel that."

We stayed in this space for about twenty minutes, playing out her memories like a movie.

"Now get a picture of Garrett today and imagine directing that affection toward him."

"I can't. It's blocked. Nothing."

This is why positive thinking strategies don't work on their own. When someone is pissed, they don't want to do that. She wasn't just mad at Garrett, she was disappointed in the whole institution of marriage and even love. Her entire life quest had been about finding love and then marriage. She was exultant on her wedding day. Now, *What a fraud,* she thought. *This is marriage. Me, at home folding clothes and cleaning bathtubs while he peruses the Internet.* She missed her college roommates. She missed getting drunk and flirting.

"Do you know what housework symbolizes to him?"

"Things he doesn't have to do."

Her flippant attitude was starting to annoy me.

"Come on. You're not being fair. Be curious about him."

"I've been married six months and already I feel taken for granted. I kind of want to get out now and find a new one."

Melissa wasn't listening to a word of my suggestions. She bulldozed forward pushing forth her dirt mound of toxic contempt. She wanted to use therapy to complain, but I can only take so many hours of indignation. Yes, therapy is about expressing thoughts and feelings, but without any evolution, it's like being at the other end of a fire hose of negative energy all day long. She showed no patience, tolerance, or understanding.

The Women on My Couch

I looked at her sitting there, blonde hair swept up in a high ponytail that revealed the sharp edges of her face, a severely squared jaw, jutting chin, and long nose adding to a harsh and intimidating demeanor. I wondered if she could sense that I didn't totally like her. And this is a truth: therapists don't always like their patients. Before our sessions, I sat for a few moments contemplating her disappointments and began to soften into compassion. I wanted to provide real empathy, but I also didn't want to collude with her in deciding her new husband was a lemon.

"I know his lack of help feels like a betrayal and it's tempting to want to punish him by leaving," I said, hinting that her idea should be taken as a fleeting impulse.

"I deserve better."

"I agree, but are you willing to explore your role in this?"

"I need to be honest with you about something." She stopped me abruptly, clearly not interested in some lecture about compromise.

"I'm attracted to someone else."

I wasn't shocked.

"He's my yoga instructor. He's so hot, in a kind of hippie way. Not the kind of guy I'd traditionally be attracted to. But he has long dark hair, tan skin, and a tall, perfectly chiseled body—and his voice is soft, yet also masculine and deep. I've had fantasies about him for a long time. (I'm sure most of the women in the class do.) I wait for that moment in class when he comes over to 'adjust' me, and he places his hands on my hips for just a little too long. I get so turned on. I swear I can feel the heat of his body, his desire. I start to fantasize that we are in a private class, and I'm wearing a low-cut top, and when he touches me, he can't resist, that he starts to move his hands across my body, that he moves closer, and he can't help but put me on the ground and fuck me."

"Do you imagine what he'd be like as a boyfriend or a husband?" I wanted to see how far this vision went.

"He's very spiritual, he's a very loving man—more evolved than most men. Able to respond to the sensitivities in a woman with great wisdom and compassion. I bet he'd know what to do with a woman in bed."

"So, this is what you're not getting in your marriage?"

"Garrett is like a primate compared to Kai. His name is Kai." She paused to smile again. "I'm not sure if I'm in love with Garrett anymore. I'm going to sign up for a private yoga class."

Melissa set this guy up to be her rescuer, an easy getaway. It's normal for crushes to happen while married, but they can get idealized. We tend to imagine them as faultless lovers who would meet our needs completely. We hardly see them as real people. Maybe hot yoga guy has IBS or still lives with his mother. Melissa seemed blinded by her own desires and not ready for self-reflection. I was concerned she would act.

I wish people told the truth at weddings. Every once in a while, some curmudgeonly uncle will grumble, "Marriage is hard work," but does anybody really know what that means? Does that uncle ever sit us down and guide us to understand that love and marriage entail patience for idiosyncrasies and *curiosity* rather than contempt? Nobody talks about a skill called frustration tolerance. Cantankerous uncles are right: marital love is straight up hard.

In my book *The Men on My Couch*—stories of men in therapy—I talk about David. He was one of my first clients, a suave womanizer, the kind who charms but never calls, the guy most women love to hate. David walked into my office and, after trying to flirt with me, asked a shockingly earnest question: "Am I capable of love?"

It was a wise question, one we should all ask before getting married. Being honest, even I was more inclined to monitor whether my partner was capable of loving me properly, ready to hand out citations for wrongdoings, such as a failure to make me tea when I was sick or to call when he was coming home late. I used to get into relationships and have a bunch of expectations—demands, really. But marriage is not an all-you-can-eat buffet. And becoming aware of that fact is like ice water to the face or being tased, or maybe both at the same time. It's a mega-consciousness-expanding moment to realize that there is much, much more to love than having someone at your behest to love and comfort you exactly how and when you want. When I learned to reorient my-self toward my own ability to love, it was one of my greatest moments of emotional freedom. (I just read this section to my husband, and he said that he is, in fact, an all-you-can-eat buffet.)

I have sat witness to many humans profoundly disappointed in the opposite sex. They blame love. Love dies. Love sucks. This makes me want to get a huge megaphone and scream:

It's not love's fault.

Love is actually pretty stable. Love doesn't deceive us. It doesn't walk away or disappear for no reason. We do.

I knew that I could guide my clients only as far as my own capacity, so I had to reconsider my own approach to love.

This question my client David posed, Am I *capable* of love, changed my life. When I reflected upon this question, I turned to someone who knew more about loving than I did. My mom. Being a stalwart for Jesus, she referred me right to the Holy Bible to read Corinthians, Chapter 13. Despite a remnant attitude of childhood resistance to religion, I dusted off my old Bible and opened it. The first line said, "Love is pa-tient." Boring. What else? I read each line impatiently.

Then it dawned on me that I didn't meet any of the criteria. Me, the serial romantic, didn't meet any of *God's* criteria for love. Corinthians tells us love is patient, kind, slow to anger and very specifically states that love is not self-seeking.

Deflated, I thought: *This is what love is?* It's not romance? It sounded like hard work. Instead of conjuring images of making love in the rain, my mind went to blue overalls and grease. The truth is, this Bible pas-sage is the most accurate depiction I've read of what love is. It's not about a series of epic movie moments; it's acceptance, compassion, un-derstanding. These are the less glamorous parts of love. The ones we ignore or overlook in favor of the fast-cars, hot-sex version. But these are the sustainable parts of love, the sturdy foundation: without them, the sweeter stuff tends to come tumbling down.

My focus had always been on how to procure love. How to be-come more lovable so that others would desire me. I would be happy, temporarily, when I was successful. So much of the euphoria of my old days came from the illusive and temporary highs of being desired.

This did not prepare me for marriage.

And now that I'm married, I am by no means an expert. It pains my ego at times to admit this, because psychologists are expected to be just that, experts. I'm sure my husband wishes more than anyone that I'd be more expert. I'd been through my own anger over domestic matters, but worse, I liked to yell about it—and then blame it on being Irish.

What I have developed over the years is a skill set, one that may be the single most important change made in my approach to relationships. I knew it would help Melissa. Again, I didn't learn these concrete elements of how to love from psychology; I learned them from Buddhism.

I go to a local center in L.A., where I take a seat on a cushion and sit silently among other people, mostly a crowd of tattooed and pierced rocker types on Melrose Avenue. We close our eyes while a teacher leads us into an attitude of loving-kindness toward whatever we're experiencing in that moment. After some time, the attention is moved away from ourselves as we're asked to contemplate the universality of our suffering by directing compassion toward all who are going through similar feelings: the person sitting next to us, the difficult people in our lives, and the strangers we encounter on the streets and in traffic.

We've all heard the old adage that you can't love until you've learned to love yourself. Buddhism emphasizes the opposite approach—loving others as the path to discovering the truth about love.

Buddhism basically defines love as wanting other people to be happy, the opposite of the American imperative, where selfhood is seen as the path to happiness. Meditative practices train the mind into a perspective of loving. I wish loving didn't have to be "trained" into my mind, that it came more naturally, but it doesn't. With practice, I can temporarily emerge from the habit of self-cherishing to other-cherishing. It's a happier place but difficult to maintain without effort. I revert back to self-absorption all the time—and I don't view this as immorality or a character flaw. From my observations of people, it's the human baseline.

The Women on My Couch

When I choose to spend time practicing loving-kindness, all of my relationships are impacted and I begin to know what those words recited in so many marriage vows actually feel like. I can *feel* the honor. I can *feel* the cherishing. And now, this word *love*, a word so trite I can't even feel it when I say it, finally reverberates through my being, an upswell of fullness in my chest, an expansive, radiant flow. Love finally feels like strength instead of insecurity.

Melissa and I began these practices together. She was about as excited as a teenager going to the mall with her parents on a Friday night. If she had pursued Kai, she didn't tell me. Each session began with ten minutes of compassion training. I asked Melissa to try loving the dishes as she washed them, loving the food she ate on them, and loving the fact that she was caring for her home. Then I had her narrate his actions out loud with a voice of kindness and empathy in place of getting judgmental. I had her imagine that he wanted the same thing as her: a happy household. We practiced wishing that for her and for him. And, finally, I had her imagine she was a target for his love. She was dubious, but she did all of it with me, and finally became open to his point of view.

"Did you find out what housework means to him?

"Yes. He didn't think taking care of the house was symbolic of equality. He saw home as a place to relax after work and looked forward to getting home to hang out with me. He said he felt abandoned by my obsessive need to clean and organize. He thought I was turning into his mother and wondered what kind of marriage he had signed up for. He was so irritated that he threw his own protest, which was to leave that plate of brussels sprouts on the floor to show me that dirty plates weren't more important than our relationship."

"How did it feel to hear that?"

"Better. He wasn't trying to subjugate me. He was just trying to relax. He claims he would do things on his own time if I didn't take over and start assigning him tasks. He's been a lot better ever since we had that conversation. He takes his plate to the kitchen, but he washes it when he feels like it."

Garrett had a right to be less focused on housework, but not to demand that she put up with his way—exactly as he wanted it—either. But this wasn't couples therapy. All I could do was give Melissa tools for marriage. I needed to be that impertinent old uncle who sits you down at the wedding to tell you what makes a marriage work: negotiating differences, compromising, allowing other perspectives, accepting idiosyncrasies, and remembering that right and wrong ways of doing anything don't matter. And most important of all, an attitude of loving-kindness.

As Melissa began to access a greater appreciation for Garrett, she softened toward him and had a more balanced perspective. Once she could see outside of the old narrative, she could allow Garrett to have his own reality.

"We had sex last night, and something weird happened. My vagina just closed up. Like literally."

Now she had vaginismus, a spontaneous muscle spasm that closes the vaginal walls. An involuntary bodily manifestation of stress, trauma, disgust, and so forth. The resentment had been cleared with Garrett and she'd felt more loving than she had in a long time, so I was curious about why her body was resisting.

Tears began to roll down her face.

"There's something I didn't tell you. I'm so embarrassed. I hired Kai for a private session and I made a move on him. I leaned in for a kiss… and he stopped me, said something about a 'loving boundary.' I feel like such an idiot and…guilty that I went that far."

Melissa had convinced herself that she was justified in looking outside the marriage because Garrett had betrayed his end of the contract by being a terrible husband. Now that she'd learned the truth about relationships—that love is conditional, and unconditional love is only a lofty moral imperative—her rationalization faded and guilt emerged.

"I feel so guilty about Kai. Should I tell Garrett?"

I never push clients to tell their partner when they've cheated. I'm not the moral police. My focus was her mental well-being. But she wanted to relieve her emotional burden by dumping the truth on him. I'd rather her do what one is supposed to do with guilt—correct the errant behavior. And that I could ride her ass about. But I didn't have to. Melissa had a renewed motivation to make therapy work. She'd became one of those studious clients who asks for homework and actually does it. She declared that she was committed to learning how to love Garrett better. Her motivation may not have been the Buddhist ideal of selflessness, but realizing a mistake and deciding to change was good enough for me. Now that she'd done some basic love practices, she was ready to move to the next step in changing her gaze: savoring.

Isabel Allende quoted a friend in her aphrodisiac cookbook *Aphrodite*, "Our obsession with variety has a lot to do with the lost gift of savoring a simple tomato." We take in tons of stimuli throughout a day, and we don't really pause on a particular sensation. Sex is an opportunity to slow down and appreciate the depth of our senses, to linger in pleasure with no goal in mind, a time to touch and actually feel each other. Allende is right, the ability to savor is a forgotten art.

I asked Melissa to try savoring Garrett, to choose one part of his body, the lower lip, a finger, an earlobe. I asked her to see and smell and feel with an attitude of appreciation, to try to connect to the essence of him that lies beyond the physical.

As I learned to slow down to perceive the beauty of another, my eyes opened with a new reverence. Without an attitude of appreciation, we treat each other in ways that are perfunctory, dehumanized, dispassion-ate, and, worst, harmful. Many of us know what it feels like when some-one treats sex as an interaction no more important than the exchange you just had with the cashier at the corner 7-Eleven. Married couples treat each other this way all the time. It's a real adjustment to look at one's husband and to see his magnificence.

"It's not easy to shift from being agitated to appreciating his eyes, but I need you to hold on to seeing the whole of him, so it's going to take practice to reprogram your thoughts. We want to keep your relationship sexualized."

"I'll try, but I wish I didn't have to try so hard."

Melissa had a good point—one that most of my clients bemoan. Maintaining interest takes serious effort. Most of us require certain conditions to be in place to get in the mood. One wants to be not tired, not busy, not bloated, not too cold, and, most of all, not annoyed with the guy. Now, what is the probability on any given day, that these criteria will all be aligned? It's like waiting for some rare moon eclipse. Perhaps it's unrealistic to demand a perfect emotional environment.

"I say we start with whatever is true in the moment. Sexualize your immediate situation and environment. Instead of limiting your arousal to when you're in a good mood or feeling pretty, this technique is learning how to eroticize every mood: sleepy, lazy, and even irritable. If he's hairy, now he's hairy hot. If you're twenty pounds over your ideal weight, now you're curvy hot. If you feel ugly, it's ugly hot. Got it?"

"How am I going to make it hot when he leaves his plates on the table? Lazy hot? Rude hot?" She laughed.

"Well, you get angry at him, right? Can anger be hot? Think of something that would turn this fight into something erotic."

"That's hard."

"Do you want to yell at him? Flirt with him? Think."

"OK, I could sit on his lap and whisper in his ear, 'Do you know how to make me happy?' And I'll look at the dish, and he will totally know what I'm talking about. Then, I will walk toward the bedroom and say, 'Let me show you what a happy woman looks like.'"

Melissa was actively *up-regulating* her sexuality, as the late Helen Singer Kaplan would say, and it was working. We'd begun with basic loving-kindness, then added the skills of sensuality, and then she was ready to add some eroticism. If I had done these out of turn, therapy would have failed. Most people don't want to get erotic with people they don't like. That's why spice-it-up books don't always work and why so many studies that measure women's desire don't give us accurate results: there's no control for hidden resentment.

I was recently asked to give a speech at my best friend's wedding. Even though I write about love, I found the task difficult because I didn't want to sound trite in a profound moment. And I didn't want to get up there and give some lecture about how marriage is WORK. Nobody wants to hear that on their wedding day. Nor did I want to give a couples therapy lecture on what makes a marriage successful. The best advice I could offer to the couple was to make a commitment to lov*ing*. When in doubt, I put my hope in this line from Corinthians, "Love never fails," and then return to my practice.

Marriage *is* a series of "inconveniences," but those moments are also opportunities for personal transformation, for marriage to be a spiritual discipline. By the end of her time with me, Melissa described the experience of loving as peaceful, warm, and full. She and Garrett had discussed the division of household duties and drew up a contract. Melissa said that she walked away from therapy with a better sense of what it means to "love, honor, and cherish." And noted that the next thing they would do on the floor would be to have sex.

Laura

They debated their belief in marriage before they did it. Should they marry if gays couldn't? Was marriage an outdated institution? Was monogamy even natural? But, ultimately, they wanted it. And three years into the marriage, they were on my couch. Laura and Brian played dodgeball on Sunday nights, drank craft beer, and had a wide circle of friends, leftist intelligentsia types. These folks had a nice life. A match made in Portlandia heaven. Or in L.A., Silver Lake heaven.

Brian had proposed an idea to Laura that he thought would be fun. A threesome. With a woman. Now, this kind of suggestion from one's husband would be outrageous and insulting to most of my female clientele, but these two ran in a crowd of convention-busting bisexual and gender-neutral friends who copulated in every possible arrangement. Laura had had girlfriends in the past, but she'd been decidedly monogamous in marriage. Before making a decision that could possibly change their relationship forever, she suggested a consultation with me.

I don't dole out direct advice on these matters. I've witnessed both positive and negative outcomes for this scenario. Mostly negative, as I am a psychologist, so my pool of references consists of people with problems. I do help patients make conscious decisions and that requires reflection on their relationship, histories, and personal motivations. The most immediately important factors are what a threesome would mean to each of them, what they would be getting out of it, and why now. However, I've found that this exploration can be dangerous.

Laura and Brian had the warm, playful presence of two people who legitimately loved spending time together. She was larger than him in form and charisma. He seemed more measured and pensive, and leaned back to let her take the lead.

"I'm open to a threesome....I want to say that I can handle it, but I've seen it ruin relationships."

Brian countered, "I've had a lot of sex in my life and it's very rare that I have romantic feelings toward anybody, as I do you. I can separate adult play from the special connection that we have. I think the probability that I will have some dangerous attraction to her is very low. The benefit is that we have a great time."

Laura and Brian were laying out their initial positions. They sat on the couch, facing each other rather than me, and held hands. Even though Laura's words were expressing some fear, her tone was unaffected, as if she were discussing what kind of takeout to get. His soft voice met hers in equal measure of cool.

Laura and Brian were friends with another married couple that had an open relationship. The woman had tried everything, from escorting to polyamory, and was encouraging Laura to try the threesome. The friend said it was a good exercise in getting over your own ego—and that once you did, it was limitless adventure. She claimed to feel very free, yet still loyal to her partner. Laura imagined herself above the restraints of common jealousy and possessiveness that tether most couples to a single mooring.

As a therapist, I witness daily how people's ideals are felled by the realities of their capacity, and I knew an attempt to transcend the ego or to control an inherently capricious impulse like Eros would pose a real risk to the relationship.

I asked Brian, "Why now?"

"Our sex is good, but sometimes a little stale. I thought if we experimented once in a while, it would be good for the relationship."

This couple was freakishly Zen in a discussion that should elicit some anxiety. They each spoke as if they had taken communication classes. They listened, empathized, and affirmed love to each other. Could they possibly be more evolved than I?

Their approach to sex was similar. They believed their love could be compartmentalized and safely sealed while they embarked on shared titillations. Both believed that attraction to other people was natural and that sharing that sexual energy was better than keeping it a secret. *But he said the sex was stale, and not even a wince from her*, I thought. I decided to prod a bit. I don't trust a lack of anxiety.

"Tell me about your sense that the sex is stale. What exactly does that feel like?" I asked Brian.

"I'm not really motivated to do it. If I'm on my computer, I'd rather do that. If a good show is on, I'd rather do that. Maybe I've watched too much porn, but regular sex isn't turning me on."

I glanced over at her for a reaction. She was slouched back on the couch with her arm over the top. She was Korean American and had her hair fixed in a 1940s-inspired roll above her forehead and wore black eyeliner that formed an exaggerated line at the corner of each eye. She looked like she was ready to dance the foxtrot.

I imagined most people would be hurt to hear that their lover was more interested in electronic devices. I wanted to ask about that, but I sensed the timing was off. I would likely get a defensive reaction.

"What's missing for you, Laura?"

"I feel like we're just masturbating together. We watch porn during sex—and don't get me wrong, it turns me on—but it's like we need a third focus of attention."

She looked down. I sensed that she was trying to hide sadness. I felt a wave of empathy for her. Why did she need to appear so above it all?

"I noticed you looking down."

"Oh—uh, just thinking."

As I'd thought, she wasn't going to let me in. She really needed to save face here. Brian interjected:

"Chemistry is missing. We have a little bit, but we made a value decision to marry each other for love, not chemistry. But I'm not resigning myself to a life without good sex; I want to push the boundaries of eroticism—with Laura. I think when you confine sex to two people, you restrain your natural impulses and creativity. There is so much more to experience than what we're doing."

He was really trying to sell me on the idea. Brian wasn't really exploring the possible impact of a threesome; he wanted me to help push the idea through. Laura and Brian had put in effort to enjoy their sex life—and it wasn't working. Their solution was to take their eroticism to the outer edges of their comfort zone. We needed to figure out if that was the right direction for them. They wanted to turn outside of the relationship for a fix, but I had a sense something was deeply wrong internally.

Laura and Brian bore the hallmarks of a couple that doesn't fight. Further, she was one of those people who smiled after every sentence. A confusing, humorless smile. I pried around for a while, looking for the hidden caches of resentment that we all harbor. Money, household responsibilities, "He's always late"—something. They didn't bite. The story was that they were perfectly compatible. They didn't express any differences. When two people need to cling rigidly to the idea that they're a flawless couple, even in front of a therapist, there is something *they* don't want to see. This made their situation a real quandary. Neither wanted to abandon the relationship because their sex wasn't hot enough. They wanted it to work. But was it possible to manufacture chemistry?

When my clients wrestle with important relationship decisions—to marry or not, to break up or not, to end an affair or not—the word "chemistry" often arises. People want to know what to do when they meet someone who is perfect on paper but the attraction is less than earth-shattering. Others lose the spark but don't want to end an otherwise good relationship either. Desire is often in conflict with our ideals.

When I ask people where the excitement comes from, I typically get some variation of "It just happens." What they do know is that they *should* have it and they're not "happy" without it—oh, and that they deserve it. Some remain single for years and despair that they can't find "it." When they do experience some electricity, they believe it's a sign that this person is special, a "soul mate." If they lose this spark, it could be cause for serious disillusionment, affairs, and even divorce. These are some pretty grave decisions for an elusive and transitory feeling most people can't even define.

What is a realistic expectation for chemistry? Should it be among the criteria for marriage? Should we be feeling it all day? How about every day? Can we expect to keep it in long-term relationships?

I think it's important to have some understanding of chemistry before making a major life decision based on its presence or absence. But most people don't want to contemplate chemistry. They just want it to happen. This idea that infatuation strikes by divine force was cherished by the ancient Greeks, though they saw it as an affliction. A capricious Eros would smite people with desire. The Greeks weren't eager to find Eros, nor did they want to marry it. Today, we are obsessed with finding the spark—to our detriment. The idea that chemistry has to be found, that it's hard to obtain, and that some special person magically possesses it leads us down the wrong path.

Given my fancy for history, I thought I would journey to another era to see how this quest for elusive chemistry was handled. I asked myself, *What was the most prurient time in human history?* Then I remembered the *Kama Sutra*. I owned a copy but didn't know where it was. This was a book that had initially put me off because half of it is dedicated to having sex with other people's wives, courtesans, servants, harems, and so on. I dismissed it as from a very male-serving, unfairly hierarchical culture. I looked around and eventually found it in my trunk buried beneath a beach umbrella and some old shoes. Opening the book was a reminder that this culture had sexual imagery weaved throughout everyday life.

When I first moved to California, my roommate and I placed the *Kama Sutra*, a large illustrated copy, and a phallic-shaped metal tool we found in the garage, next to each other on the coffee table in our living room. Then, when we'd have dates, we'd watch to see which item they'd pick up. A kind of Rorschach test for overt versus covert sexuality. Almost nobody picked up the *Kama Sutra*. Too bad, because it featured some pretty awesome depictions of graphic sex acts in the architecture, pottery, paintings, and temples—art that celebrated homosexuality, group sex, transgender people, and even bestiality. This was a seriously sexually amped period, and I figured that if anyone knew how to create some electricity, it was these folks.

When I revisited the *Kama Sutra*, I realized that this 527-page manual is part of a series of books on living a sophisticated life, not just a bunch of pictures of contorted sex positions. Compiled around the fourth century CE by a philosopher named Vatsyayana, in a period of cultural flourishing, the book captures an era in which urban sophisticates aspired to three aims of life: ethics, material success, and eroticism. Yes, eroticism—not sex—was a primary virtue and one of the central points of a civilized existence.

Erotic training was an important part of society in the age of the *Kama Sutra*. Men were trained in "amorous approaches"—sixty-four of them, to be exact. Women were taught the art of conversation; how to decorate, dance, and sing; various arts and crafts; how to dress and bejewel themselves; magic; storytelling; the "art of cheating"; poetry; even metal- and woodworking. My point is that these people didn't sit around waiting to be smitten by some external force; nor did they haplessly search through a vast number of strange faces. They believed that chemistry was cultivated through practice. My clients are inclined to balk at this idea. They want to be enchanted, seduced, and given over to a spell. Before you get turned off by the work implied in the word "practice," let me share, in my interpretation, the details of "the practice" outlined in the *Kama Sutra*.

First, there is a room, separate from the rest of the house, with nothing in it but a bed, flowers, and incense. The gentleman takes a bath, dresses in fine attire, and gathers his friends and servants to enter this "chamber of love." He sits down next to the woman, offers her a drink, and begins to make small talk, telling funny stories. He regales her with riddles and gossip, slowly interjecting "indecent" or "vulgar" themes in order to arouse her. Then music and song begin, and they may get up and dance. Afterward, they talk about art, and he encourages her to drink more. As he is chatting, he strokes her hair, and while she is distracted, he undoes her robe in the area between her thighs. He may show her some phallic drawings.

Eventually, he gives her an oil of flower essence, which he applies to her body, and serves her betel, which is a cue for everyone else to leave the room. He then "tears off her robe," and they begin to have sex. He chooses positions that will provide the most pleasure, given her and his body type and the size of their sex organs (information he has gathered ahead of time). When they finish, they are both to go to the bathroom and clean up in separate quarters, then return to the bed, where he will rub sandalwood paste all over her body. He will also pat fine powder on any bruises incurred by their aggression. He puts his arms around her, talks to her sweetly, and offers her "grilled meats, drinks of ripe fruit juice.… Then at their ease, they drink sweet liquor, while chewing from time to time sweet or tart things." Later, they climb to the terrace on the roof to enjoy the moon and stars and continue their pleasant conversation.

This ritual may sound contrived—and most of my clients have an aversion to anything contrived—but the *Kama Sutra* was all about using a script. There was no expectation for spontaneity; being in "the mood" was not a prerequisite. A ritual circumvents these two modern expectations about sex.

Most Americans will not have time for this (at least not every night); but rather than the perfunctory duty sex Americans know all too well, the ritual creates an atmosphere of superlative sensuality. Although it's a routine, this custom sounds anything but boring as it mixes art, aggression, food, and dance.

I will concede that this ritual alone probably wouldn't get a woman turned on to just anybody, and they did first match people according to what was considered important for their getting along: temperament, astrology, and the size of sex organs. The *Kama Sutra* states that "true erotic satisfaction" is established via routine sexual practice by people who share an "ordinary attraction." Which seems to mean that there is compatibility; just like my clients and their lovers who are lacking only the dizzying initial physical attraction. According to the *Kama Sutra*, it is practice that causes love and desire to grow over time. Laura and Brian could be classified in the ordinary attraction category given that they were highly compatible with a mild physical attraction.

So how do these ancient date nights differ from Brian's attempts at spicing it up, like porn viewing, role-play, and threesomes? The *Kama Sutra* rituals have plenty of props, between the musicians and phallic drawings and all, but in the end, they served to enhance a connection between the lovers. This was a very different use of props from Brian and Laura's—which enhanced their eroticism, but not necessarily toward each other. They were stuck in a parallel play situation, where the focus of their respective erotic attentions was the third stimulus. Inspired by the *Kama Sutra*, I asked them to create their own version of a ritual at home. A threesome is a risky option, because it's hard to anticipate the emotional consequences, so I wanted them to try directing their Eros at each other to see what would happen. This would also tell me something about the truth of their bond.

Laura and Brian were enthusiastic about the idea. They went home and made a bed of pillows on the floor of their living room, lit candles, spread out bowls of grapes, nuts, and sliced papaya and mango, and poured white wine. She wore only a long, gold necklace and draped scarves around her body. They played sitar ambient music, lit incense, and read a few erotic poems. They took their time exploring each other's bodies. Laura said that she felt relaxed and joyful as he began to enter her—then he lost his erection.

Laura was dispirited. She realized that when all distractions were removed, she alone couldn't turn him on like she used to. When she described this to me, I could sense the shame she felt in her femininity as she presented her body, naked and exposed, while his body, which couldn't lie, mercilessly rejected her. Laura was not a beauty by conventional standards, not that Brian would have preferred a conventional beauty. She wasn't voluptuous in all the right places. She was a real woman, and she was sexual.

I suspected that his reaction wasn't about her desirability. In most cases, it's a reflection of his inner experience; his body revealing something he perhaps doesn't want to acknowledge. After hearing about the failed homework assignment, I split them up and talked to them each alone for twenty minutes. If I kept them together, I knew they wouldn't be completely open and honest. And experience had shown me that if I confronted their inauthenticity first, they were likely to turn on me instead of each other. I bypassed that problem for the time being. I took Laura to my waiting room and sat down with Brian.

"Close your eyes and go back to that moment. Allow yourself to feel it."

"OK, got it."

"Imagine moving toward her, looking in her eyes, moving into her body. What comes up?"

"I see her, but there is a nothingness, a void. Um, then I feel weird about that, and I want to move or change position so I don't look at her."

"Stay there—what will happen if you do?"

"A heavy, claustrophobic feeling. I want out of there."

His demeanor, which tended to be detached and intellectual, had kept me feeling pushed back. I was glad to be dipping into a real feeling.

"Do you have daydreams about 'getting out of there'?" He paused and furrowed his brow, considering whether he really wanted to answer my question.

"Yes. I hate admitting this, but sometimes I fantasize about having an affair. But I don't really want to do that. I want to be in the relationship. I just question whether it was right to marry my best friend or if I should have waited until I met someone who blew my mind. But I've never met anybody that made me feel that way. I wonder if it's me. I'm a nice guy, I want passion, but I don't feel anything deeply. I'm pretty much in the same state every day, a baseline affability, mild annoyances here and there, but nothing moves me to tears or makes me want to bound with joy. I mean, if my dog dies, the next day I'm in that same pleasant mood."

Brian was a nice, normal guy. He seemed to be the kind of man who'd go buy you tampons or stay the course through a cancer diagnosis with quiet patience and loyalty. But inside his being, each high or low was muted. He couldn't surrender into the deep, couldn't fall into an experience, without a drowning sensation. There was no pleasure in abandon. He was fine, as long as he swam near the surface. I see so much of this in practice, placid people whose only discomfort is an emptiness, a vague sense of alienation.

"So, do the porn and strip clubs help you to get some breathing room?"

"We'll be in bed together and I'll fantasize about Laura with another woman or I'll remember a video I really like, and my mind is on tits, lots of them, rubbing up against each other, against me, me fucking their tits. Sometimes Laura looks at me, and I can see in her eyes some focused intensity. I don't really know what that is. It freaks me out."

Brian also confided that since they'd moved in together, he saw his friends less on his own, that they did everything as a couple, and that his independent sense of self was fading. To top it off, she was starting to talk about having children. I'd been wondering why he had suggested the threesome at this point in the relationship—and now it was beginning to make sense.

Brian presented his point of view in a way that was overly strident and now it was becoming clear that it served a purpose. He needed the space that a spiritually and emotionally meaningless threesome would provide. He thought that erotic intelligence meant separating love and lust; that the former would be safe while the latter was toyed with. He thought he could love one woman and lust for another. But I wasn't so sure that compartmentalization, a common defense of the psyche in trauma situations, was going to be as easy as he imagined. Compartmentalizing is a form of splitting, a forced denial of some charged and intolerable energy. And therapists know that when people try to hide things away in the hidden crevices of consciousness, the stuff always finds its way back. Love and lust need not be split. The internal rumblings of dissonance will shout against the repression. The mind prefers harmony, and the split between love and lust is an illusion, a false dichotomy. The rude, aggressive impulses of animal lust are not necessarily incongruous with love.

I had to honor his privacy, so I wasn't able to tell Laura about his concerns. I brought her in next.

"What's missing for you in this sexual relationship?"

"I feel an emptiness. It's hard to explain, but it makes me want to cry. Like something deep in my soul wants to wail out loud, but I don't know why."

"See if you can remember the last time you felt like that."

"OK. The other day, I was watching Brian with our friends, and he was being really witty, and I had this moment of being proud he was my husband. It turned me on. When we got home, I started undressing him. We went over to the couch and started our sort of routine way of touching, and I started to feel sad."

"Describe 'sad.'"

"I don't know—it's like he can't see me or doesn't want to. I somehow feel alone."

Across clients, I have seen people try to articulate this ineffable hunger. It was a yearning beyond lust, beyond quotidian ego gratifications, and beyond even their ideas of love. It was the exasperated roar of a soul unseen. I wondered if their mutual decision to separate sex and love, to separate mind and body, created an unseen rending that upended some natural harmony of the sexual universe.

"Umm…What did you do?"

"I went through the motions and eventually I faked an orgasm."

"Why?"

"It's like this automatic reaction that I'm barely conscious of, but if I had to put words to it, it would be: *I don't want him to be mad at me.* I don't want him to cheat on me. I know he gets restless. He's not the kind of guy to settle for a mediocre life, in or out of the bedroom. I want to keep it hot, and so I do anything he wants—I even suggest it. I do like it though, I like that we're open to things, but there is some emotional chasm there that I can't put my finger on."

When I try to assess the state of any couple, I always think of a closeness–distance continuum and imagine where they lie. A couple that is too close may need to try sexual activity that gives them distance. Couples with too much distance may need more connected sex. However, the individuals who make up these couples are often not in the same place. Just as Laura yearned with the violence of a restless sea, Brian was desperately looking for a lifeboat. This was going to be difficult for me to integrate.

What happens at this moment of collision is extremely revelatory about the relationship status. Do they talk about the difference? Fight? Remain silent? They played perfect too many sessions and now that I had split them up, I got the truth. I asked each of them why they couldn't do this in the couples session. Both acknowledged their patterns. Laura tended to capitulate. Her parents fought in front of her, and she thought if she was good, which meant compliant and agreeable, that her parents would get along better and that they wouldn't divorce. Brian described his single mother as disorganized and anxious. He, her only child, stepped into a husband-like role with her. Brian compulsively needed to control his environment, always making sure he got what he wanted, and, in the process, failed to let others be who they were. The subtle demand—which he didn't dare express—was, "You better be what I want, because I am dependent on you to feel happy." Laura largely did everything his way, and both were more or less at peace. When couples like Laura and Brian come to therapy, their reluctance to express difference becomes evident quickly and must be addressed or therapy stalls.

The withholding of their mutual disappointment was a clue to their sexual problem. I gathered from Laura that after they had married, the relationship subtly and insidiously moved from a place driven by joy to one motivated by fear. They avoided confrontations and thought they were successful for never fighting. This wasn't stability—it was stagnation.

Dependency in relationships is a phenomenon particular to modern living. We tend to couple off and, like Laura and Brian, live far away from our families, with only a few friends. I went hiking with a dear friend at Runyon Canyon, an L.A. city park that has been declared America's sexiest hiking trail. Locals refer to it as a dog park with some models running around. I was lamenting to my friend that in order to hang out, we have to make a "play date." There are no more spontaneous visits or late night talks about boys. We only live twelve miles away from each other—which means an hour driving time. This decreases the chances even further of making a date, limiting our time to once a week at best. To maintain the feeling of a community in an adult life takes serious effort. Otherwise, you simply meet up over brunch twice a month and have little to talk about. The narrowness of adult social networks puts extra pressure on a couple to meet too many emotional needs. This one person is responsible for too many needs—and, of course, the heaviness of that causes boredom. Then to fix the problem, we think we need edgy experiences to create vitality again.

Threesomes existed in the ancient world. In fact, members of the oldest religion in India, Shaivism, built temples full of reliefs with sexual unions of threes, fours, fives, and even animals fucking, sucking, and stripping in every possible arrangement. This was six thousand years before Christ, and these folks were super kinky. But the meaning of these interactions was symbolic, purposeful, and highly spiritual. Themes of honor, worship, and a divine order of energy imbued this behavior, not titillation for bored people.

The *Kama Sutra* has something to offer us for the problem of dependency that tends to occur in any domestic context. The writers of this text understood that passion requires expression. They took what most modern Americans are afraid of, like anger or difference, and created an erotic outlet for it. Conflict was viewed as normal, not something to shy away from, and there is a script for how to fight "appropriately." They celebrate the natural tension in relationships by giving detailed instructions on how to bite and scratch and strike. The *Kama Sutra* even mentions the necessity of post-lovemaking attacks of anger and the infamous "love quarrels"—all designed to enhance passion. It's notable that these love quarrels are described in the chapter dedicated to "erotic games" and the induction of desire. I will describe below, again in my own words, how to fight sexy.

The Women on My Couch

Once a woman's passion has intensified because her partner has been working his sixty-four moves on her, she may become easily jealous or angry when he disagrees with her. But instead of trying to be agreeable or more perfect, she "weeps with rage, her head and body trembling, seizes the boy by his hair so as to hit him, then throwing herself onto the ground, she tears off her necklaces and jewels." The author then interjects for the guy, "never should he mock the girl lying on the ground." He is instructed to lovingly pick her up and put her back on the bed, speaking sweet nothings. And she is to begin beating him again: "Raising his face, she strikes with her feet at his arms, his face, his breast….Then she goes as far as the door and, sitting on the threshold, weeps waterfalls of tears." She is never to leave, or it's understood that she can't come back. The symbolism of standing at the door is that she could leave, but she doesn't. He then comes over, *not fearing her anger at all,* takes her into his arms, and now they make some serious love. That's the erotic game. It has several variations and has inspired many poems and stories in India.

If a woman behaved this way today, a guy would probably think, *This chick is psycho.* Psychotherapists would concur and likely diagnose her with borderline personality traits. Their little love quarrel sounds extreme to us today, but this was part of civilized behavior at the time. However, this scene wasn't one of wanton violence and hysterics. There was meaning to this drama—it was a theater in which they could play with all of the intense feelings that accompany love. Rather than be afraid of vulnerability, as we are today, they gave it poetry. They understood the inherent aggression in any relationship and found a way to sexualize it rather than subdue it. One of my male clients called this "The Perverted Argument."

The qualities it takes to sustain libido are different from what most expect. Lust isn't all about the soft and fuzzies of intimacy, empathy, and tenderness. When a frustrated client told me that she "wants to be ravaged" by her husband—she was onto something. Unlikely qualities such as aggression, audacity, courage, and leadership are essential for passion.

116

Brian and Laura came back in, and finally, there was a shift. They sat next to each other. He was smiling at me, with his arm around her, and her body was stiff.

"We tried it. We had a threesome," Brian declared.

Wow, they haven't fully discussed it yet, I thought. That was the reason they came in…to discuss.

"Laura initiated it. I took her with me on a business trip for three days, and she found this event called a 'first-base party.' Laura walked up to this girl and invited her to come home with us. I had to rent a room in the city on the fly, and we took her there. Then after, we were able to leave. It was an amazing night…so amazing…"

Brian was grinning, facing Laura with a loving countenance, holding her hand. I turned my gaze toward Laura and studied her face.

"How was it for you?"

"Great."

And that was all she had to say. Her lip quivered through that phony smile I'd become accustomed to seeing at the end of each sentence. Laura was in pain, yet trying to hide it. Now was the time. I had to stop this.

"So, you both had the same exact reaction," I said, aligning with the charade.

"Laura, tell me what was so great about it?"

She burst into tears. Brian pulled away, looking surprised.

"What's wrong? You initiated it—I thought you were down," he said.

She hesitated for a long time. I felt tempted to say something, but I stayed silent; I wanted the pressure to be on her to come forth.

"I did have a good experience—I did." She struggled, shame seeming to rein her in.

"It was just harder than I thought to…uh…uh…witness how excited he got about her."

He jumped in. "I was excited about you too."

"I don't think I've ever seen you that turned on. I saw the look on your face when you saw her naked body. It was ravenous, and the way you touched her so hungrily, you were giving her everything I've ever wanted. I don't understand why that couldn't be me." She turned away and silenced herself.

I looked over at him. He looked compassionate. He started to jump in and rescue her, but I put my hand up to stop him.

"Laura, try not to stop yourself. What else do you need to say?"

"I have nothing rational to say."

"Brian, can we let her be irrational for a minute? Do you think you could tolerate that?"

"Yes."

We looked at her. She flashed me a dirty look. Finally, the nice-girl façade was unraveling.

"I feel like I want to hide, to run away because I don't turn you on. I'm not hot because I'm familiar? Because I live with you and I do loving things for you like fold your fucking socks? It's not fair—why don't you look at my body like that? I hate your eyes. I'll never look at them again without seeing that sparkle in them, that desire that was for her."

Brian grabbed her chin and looked her in the eye. "I want you, and that's why I'm here. We don't ever have to do that again. It's meaningless to me. It was just lust—it's you that I love. Why can't you understand the difference?"

He looked at me as if for help in explaining the difference, but I nodded to Laura.

"It doesn't feel separate to me, Brian. Maybe my mind is not as sophisticated as yours. I don't think my heart and vagina are separate, and I don't want to force their separation either. You either love me with all of your being or not all."

She was shouting at him. He looked concerned for her in the way one looks at a screaming child.

"God, why do women have to make sex so precious? It's a carnal act. Why is it some grand test of my love to you? I do love you. I'm right here with you every day, walking through life."

"Because I can't feel you. During sex, I can't feel you at all. Your skin is cold, your eyes are vacant. *I'm* bored. How about that?" she pushed.

"It's not that I don't love you, Laura. It's marriage. I feel lost, trapped—I don't know. Marriage is fucking lonely sometimes."

He looked a little scared for the first time. She sat silent.

"I feel the same way."

"This is the first time I've seen real, alive feelings between the two of you," I said. "I want you each to close your eyes. Take a breath. Now, sitting with these emotions, I want you each to imagine how you would express these feelings to the other—through sex."

Brian and Laura were having a crisis of meaning. Was sex special? Or was it simply bodies experiencing pleasure? Further, their personal issues of loneliness and life purpose were weaving into their sex life. Both of them were stolid and cerebral, but they couldn't think their way out of this dilemma. To draw out more primitive feeling states, I assigned nonverbal homework. Their task was to follow what their bodies wanted: holding, grabbing, crying, biting, hair pulling, kissing, and so on.

Freud's idea of two drives—lust and aggression—is a useful way to think about relationships. Known as *Eros* and *Thanatos*, both drives together are thought to make a person whole. So, if aggressive instincts are buried, then we have a sappy, boring, half-authentic affair. Too much Eros, and you get what Freud called *libidinal regression*. Basically, this means that a person avoids his or her own sexual aggression by reverting to a childlike state of wishing for cuddling, succor, nurturing. Too much Thanatos and you get sadistic, impersonal, exploitive sex.

There has to be room for the very natural feelings that come up in any relationship: frustration, anger, irritation, and even sadism. These feelings can be expressed and harnessed into passion. It makes sense that people in relationships want to avoid feeling aggressive. People don't want to hurt each other and don't want to threaten the bond—for obvious reasons. Further, spiritual and political ideals remind us that we should be operating in Eros: be nice, be good, love one another, and so on. As an experiment, I once tried to be pure Eros. For months, I did daily Buddhist-based loving-kindness practices—and they were effective in transforming me into a more loving person—but I felt like a failure when I still wanted to flick off all the rude drivers on L.A.'s 101 Freeway. I realized that I wasn't a hypocritical peddler of love; I had simply forgotten Thanatos.

Anger serves us. It gets us to take action: to protect ourselves, set boundaries, demand respect. Anger helps us to be not a doormat but a solid person. It's a source of confidence. Penetration requires some level of aggression—and so does telling a man what to do. It takes fearlessness to have sex with our eyes open, to be present, to talk and share fantasies in real time, expressing a full range of feelings from love to aggression.

The next time Laura and Brian came in, it was one of those days of rare clarity, when the smog is gone and the grandeur of the surrounding mountains stand in sharp relief, a glimpse of beauty that only happens after rain—an apt metaphor for the emotional clearing that happens after the release of resentment. They talked about what had happened when they went home after that dramatic previous session.

"We went home and made love," Laura said. "I cried the whole time, and he was kissing the tears on my cheek. He was so tender, I thought my heart would break. It was the first time in a long time that we were just there with each other in the moment."

Brian concurred. "It felt good to feel something, even if it was bittersweet."

"Laura, it took a while for these feelings to come out," I observed.

"I was embarrassed that I couldn't deal with the threesome. I wanted so badly to be cool."

Laura thought she'd been defeated because she'd experienced anger and jealousy—emotions for people less evolved, less in control of themselves.

"So once you're OK with the fact that these feelings exist, rationally or irrationally, you can bring them to sex, allowing the feeling to be a constant expression of who you are or where you are. It can infuse the moment with some of the aliveness you're both looking for. Desire isn't static."

"What if I don't have anything to express? What if my mood is neutral?" asked Brian, knowing it would be a challenge for him to access emotion. He'd still rather focus on physical sensation.

"Then you can create. Try the ritual you guys did before. I'm sure it will feel different now that you've cleared the air. Or try one of your other erotic preferences. I'm sure that will feel different now."

"We did a lot of talking about marriage," Laura said. "It's not the same with my friends as when I was single. I used to live in an apartment full of people, and there was always fun and spontaneous talking—and now I have to make adult play dates. And everybody has their schedules, and kids. Life is kind of boring."

"Rather than blame this on marriage, I think this was a wake-up call for you guys to take action. Brian did the right thing by declaring the sex was stale. So many people never say a word about that. They either just accept it or they're afraid to say it, so change never happens."

How do you keep someone sexualized when you share space? This is quite a popular question in therapy. In the absence of seduction training, love chambers, and the full-on pomp of the ancient world, how do we create a modern life that supports a constant, simmering eroticism? There are nights when you don't want to wear something sexy. You want sweatpants. You want rest. The goal is not to be sexy all the time, cleaning the dishes wearing a corset or vacuuming nude wearing only heels (though these are both sexy ideas). We've got to let go of this ideal that sets us all up to fail. Quality sex, once per week, is better than quantities of crap sex.

The *Kama Sutra* rituals offer an avenue for creative expression. Knowing how to paint or tell stories was a central part of the process; the ritual even prescribes a pause to discuss art. I love that. It's an ancient concept, in more than one country by the way, that creativity and libido mutually generate each other—a connection that isn't made today. Art and sex were part of the same force.

Laura and Brian's strength was they were willing to try anything—their focus was simply misdirected. They had gotten pretty disconnected, but I had faith that they would pull through and find their way to a richer experience. Laura and Brian were figuring out how to be married, how to fight, and how to negotiate differences. They were creating the space necessary for more intensity to happen. In their short time with me, I saw no flame between them, but I did see possibility. Whether you begin a relationship with chemistry or not, there will always be some loss of it to grieve. The initial euphoria is fleeting, but eroticism persists; it just changes form over time. As Laura and Brian grow as a couple, their desire can flow along with it.

"We decided we're not going to do any more threesomes for now, but we're leaving the possibility open for the future," Laura explained. "We also decided we're not going to have a baby right now, but we'll leave that open too."

"Our focus will be on creating a marriage that breathes. We realized that we need more space and more friends," said Brian.

"And we're planning a trip to Costa Rica," added Laura.

Tara

I've been living in California for six years now, and I'm well into my forays outside of traditional psychology. Sitting in my dining-room-turned-home-office, a room that makes my husband blush when he brings colleagues over for a drink, I'm surrounded by a mess of books: illustrated copies of Indian temples covered in orgy reliefs, advice from porn stars, art from the Japanese floating world, and photographs of topless Minoan paintings. There are shelves dedicated to erotica and erotic poetry, favorite pages ripped out and plastered across the wall.

Little by little, my explorations have been turning into results in therapy. Clients participate in a range of creative, often made up on the spot, homework assignments, everything from sitting naked in front of a mirror to hiring one's husband as a houseboy to clean shirtless. They push the edges of the familiar, feeling the exhilaration of new territory, challenging the limits of their personalities and relationships.

Not every avenue I pursued collecting this cache turned out to be some new cure-all. Some of it fell flat and some was corny. In the beginning, just like my clients, I didn't know where to turn for inspiration. Even the phrase "sexual exploration" conjured the clichés of kissing another girl while drunk at a bar, buying a vibrator, or trying out bondage, all of which are fine avenues, but I was bored with pop culture. However, the intersection of ancient traditions and real life has not always gone smoothly for my clients.

Mark came in alone at first. He told me that he'd like to want sex more than a beer, or his computer, or brushing his teeth. Contrary to popular belief, many times it's the man with a low sex drive, and the woman is left agitated and horny. Mark said he'd lost all urges to have sex, alone or with his wife. And as the expert, I was expected to install said urge. A tall order. Much of therapy is focused on alleviating unwanted feelings, depression, anxiety, and so forth. But in the case of attraction, people want me to help them to conjure a *wanted* sensation. That hope casts me in the role of a feelings magician, manufacturing something out of nothing. Mark continued:

"She thinks that when I see her naked body, I should be turned on. But I'm not, it takes more than that."

He didn't say that in front of her, thank God. But he did tell his wife Tara that he wanted "more excitement from her" during sex. To which she replied, "Alright, what would you like me to do?" He explained that he didn't want her to *do* anything in particular, "just *be* more passionate."

I asked him to bring Tara to the next session. As I guided them into my office, I made my usual small talk to warm her up, but she seemed impatient. I detected an accent, grounded, guttural. I guessed at her origin and she helped me along. "Swiss German."

She sat down, crossed her arms and legs, and then faced toward him expectantly, as if to say, *OK, why are we here?*

Tara had an incredulous look on her face. I wondered what he had told her about why she was coming to therapy with him. Perhaps she was bracing for an unwanted revelation, an affair, or a breakup. Maybe she was skeptical of therapists. I decided to ask before proceeding.

"Tara, what's your understanding of why you're here today?"

"He didn't tell me he was in therapy until this morning. He said he's here because he doesn't want to have sex with me. I'm already painfully aware of that. I don't understand why I need to be dragged in to hear all about that." She kept her gaze on him.

"I'd like us to figure this out together," Mark chimed in.

"This is your problem. But, look," she softened, "I'm willing to help you out."

I asked if she understood his request to "be more passionate."

"I love sex. I want to have it every day. He's the one that turns it down."

"You treat me like a machine. I can't get an erection on demand," he escalated.

"I dress up for you. I do foreplay. I don't know what else you want me to do. Most guys I've been with will just take off my clothes and fuck me. But Mark never does that," she said, looking at me as if telling on him.

"I need to feel more connected."

"I don't know what you mean by that," she said, rolling her eyes.

"I want sex to feel transcendent. I want it to move me."

"We're married. Be realistic."

"Tara, you think you're giving me some gift by wanting sex every day. You make sex banal," he complained.

"Oh really? What are you doing about that? I'm lucky if you take your socks off. I have made so many suggestions: porn, strip clubs— even a nudist resort—and you rejected every idea."

"All of that feels hollow."

"Oh my God! What do you want? Do you know how many of our friends' husbands don't get any sex? You have a wife who wants to have sex with you! Can you help him?" She looked at me.

"It's hard to explain. I feel like she's having sex 'at me' instead of 'with me.' During sex, I feel lonely."

"What? Do you want me to stare in your eyes the whole time? That's real fucking hot. Missionary, eye staring. Can we say 'I love you' in each other's ear too?" she said sarcastically.

"What if I did want that? Why do I have to feel embarrassed to ask for it?"

Mark and Tara were on two totally different planes, orbiting in proximity but out of touch, giving their sex an autistic quality. I needed to learn more about where they were each coming from rather than taking their explanations at face value. He seemed to be having a crisis of spirit, seeking the numinous. She was more practical, into the physical realm. Weary from her lack of attunement, lack of understanding, of her mocking, Mark raised the stakes.

"I don't want to live like this for the rest of my life. I don't know if I can stay in this relationship. I feel dead inside."

"You feel uninspired in general." She waived her hand dismissively. "You have writer's block. You don't want to do anything or hang out with anybody. Don't make this existential crisis you're having *my* fault."

She had his number. Mark was a bit of a clod. An aspiring screenwriter, he stayed at home during the day and had a disheveled appearance—even by L.A. standards, where the casual look is actually the product of significant thought and effort. He was more depressed recluse than relaxed hipster. He had curly brown hair that had grown outward Malcolm Gladwell style and a pot belly from drinking. Yet he still loved to say things like "She's gained a little weight since she had our kid. I'm not attracted to her anymore." I interpreted this as pure projection of his own slovenliness and let him know it. Rarely do guys say that to me, by the way, unless they're looking for someone to blame. Also, it makes me want to shoot nails out of my eyeballs.

"Tell her how much you've been drinking," charged Tara.

"It's gone from a beer every night to three. Not that big of a deal. Yes, it's increased as our sex life has gone down, since our son was born."

"Don't blame your libido issues on Connor. This is a cop-out. Blame it on the alcohol. Blame it on yourself."

I wondered what purpose the alcohol was serving, what he wanted to feel or not feel. The single loudest complaint among all of my clients over the years, across the settings I've worked in and the cities I've lived in, is a lack of feeling. Passion is what people want—but often they can't articulate it; they just know something is missing. The experience they're yearning for is, indeed, hard to define, a gestalt difficult to break down into its component parts. The longing for this illusive force is not just coming from the repressed folks. I've had swingers and sex workers and all kinds of kinky virtuosos who struggle with a lack of feeling as well. Because my clients are aware of its absence, yet unclear about how to cultivate its presence, there is a great deal of confusion about how to stay fulfilled in relationships. Even in my psychology training, there was little mention of passion. As a result, I've been collecting the bits and pieces that comprise the essence of what people really want.

One truth is that passion cannot be demanded. Or willed. Its subtle energies are cultivated. As part of my education, I turned to erotic art. I read poetry and stories, and I began to analyze why certain pieces stayed with me for days, why some, and not others, lingered on in dreams and fantasies. The best erotic books and movies withhold sex itself as long as possible; their authors understand that the *possibility* of sex is sexier than the act itself. They want the audience begging for it, not having it thrown in their face gratuitously, and without context.

The possibility of sex contains uncertainty. Maybe it'll happen, maybe it won't. It's in that uncertain space that wanting grows. Consider the contemporary popularity of vampire fiction: it isn't the garlic cloves or dirt-filled coffins that turn people on, it's the ambiguity, the flattery, and the danger. The vampire wants the mortal woman because there's something special about her. He loves her, but he could kill her, too. Wanting meets resistance and existential threat—an old conflict that tends to strike a chord. Daily sexual demands take away the uncertainty.

Tara's approach left no room for tension building. She harbored the belief that they must have sex daily or there's a problem with the relationship. A "should": we *should* be having or wanting sex every day, or we're not living up to the American ideal of the highly sexual life. Yet, it's not real. The average American married couple has sex once per week. Nor is daily sex necessary for a fulfilling relationship, and such pressure only makes people think they're inadequate. I decided upon an experiment. I told Mark and Tara to take sex off the table.

"Now, we're never going to have sex," she said dryly.

I assigned them instead to sit and gaze into each other's eyes for twenty minutes, a technique that a colleague into Tantra had taught me. Soul-gazing, he called it. Both chuckled.

"Humor me, guys."

When I first arrived from New York, I didn't have the clientele to rent my own full-time office, so I did what most therapists with small caseloads do. I sought another therapist to rent from. I'd found a soft-spoken, bearded gentleman, late fifties, who also specialized in sex therapy. I was hoping to consult or begin a mentorship, even a friendship. With his tunic shirts and linen slacks, he looked like a cross between Freud and a yogi. He was very welcoming and had invited me out to dinner to chat about our practice. I was delighted. He was much more experienced, and I plumbed his mind for tips on issues that baffled me at the time.

He told me that he practiced Tantra. I thought, *That's right, I am so in California now.* His tone was cool and self-assured, leaving me feeling naïve for my initial impulse to dismiss it as New Age fluff. He explained that Tantra is a sexual-spiritual practice that honors the divinity in our bodies and sexuality. Penises, breasts, vaginas—are all thought to be sacred. There are parties, called *pujas*, where participants "create a sacred space" to practice their spirituality. There are red parties, in which the guests are nude or partially so, and white parties with clothes on. The parties are structured by rituals. Men and women are paired up with a member of the opposite sex. They breathe together, then touch—with intention and honor. After, there may be a snack. And a chance to chat.

My new landlord invited me to a white party. I said yes. I would go as an observer, perhaps a participant if I felt comfortable. I hated knowing that there was a whole world of sexual wisdom that I wasn't privy to. The day of the party, he proposed that we meet at the office in advance so he could teach me about Tantra—privately. I wasn't sure what he had in mind. *Did he want to touch me? That would be weird.* I didn't even want to ask since I was in the position of renting from him. I told him that I'd meet him at the party.

I arrived at a suburban house in an upper-middle-class, trendy neighborhood. I walked into a room full of people of various ages and ethnicities. There was incense burning, candles flickering, and those little Nepalese flags hanging across the living room. I saw my colleague across the room. I walked over and said hello briefly, but he was aloof, leaving me to fend for myself rather than making introductions. He seemed eager to chat with an attractive blonde who looked about his age.

I walked tepidly into the room full of people. I gazed over at a small cluster of individuals with tripped-out looks of kindness on their faces, all loving smiles and empty eyes, and then headed for the snack table. I scanned the room and noticed a disproportionate number of men. Mostly middle aged, many with little ponytails and eager friendliness. We were called to sit down, and as the group gathered in a circle, I took a seat along with them—even though I wasn't sure if I wanted any of those guys to touch me in a sacred way. First we were asked to simply move our bodies around in any way that "felt right" to loosen up. Then there was a guided meditation to "expand" our sexual energy. Then we all opened our eyes and were asked to massage the shoulders of the person next to us, creating a big circular, group massage orgy. I felt embarrassed; perhaps I was fending off an eroticism that felt threatening. Then we took turns, talking-stick style, sharing our experiences of the meditation. I remained silent.

The ideals of Tantra were sublime, but the ritual felt forced and awkward in practice. The puja was over and people began breaking up, talking informally and pairing off, some to private rooms. Oral sex may be viewed as an act of worship—an awesome way to think of it—but did I want to practice body worship with the ponytailed, pock-marked guy in a Hawaiian shirt who started to corner me with insistent conversation? I looked for my landlord, who ignored me throughout, and saw him walking down the hall with the blonde. I decided to make a run for it.

Relieved to be back in my apartment, but provoked by the experience, I sat down and started taking notes. I thought back to what initially drove me to seek out other perspectives. It was my first set of clients back in New York. I'd tried to prescribe what every new therapist is taught: the Masters and Johnson technique of turn-taking touching. One person touches the full body of the other, while the receiver focuses on the sensation of touch. The premise was to get people out of their heads and into the physical pleasure. Clients hated it. I was taught to view their reactions as "resistance" and to persuade them to continue, analyzing their defense mechanisms. Clients called it boring, mechanical, predictable. How could they have such fury at relaxing into pleasure? The exercise seemed to emphasize their lack of feeling for each other. Instead of making them horny, they felt the terror of realizing that their love was dead.

The touching rituals of the Tantra party weren't that different from the Masters and Johnson touching exercises, yet the participants found them much more appealing. These other approaches I'd been discovering, from Taoism to the *Kama Sutra*, offered a missing link: *meaning*. Modern sex therapy doesn't get that meaning matters. Many sexologists are focused on anatomy, enhancing orgasms, STD education, toys, and lube—many weirdly fascinated with lube. They all want to recommend the best lube, to display their erudition about the finest ingredients making up lube. All of this is fine, except it's not what people want to talk about in therapy. Nobody asks me about the location of their G-spot or what's the best vibrator. What they do want to talk about is much more ineffable.

Tara called and asked if she could come in by herself. She was wearing her workout clothes, still sweaty from her boxing class. I noticed that she was much more fit than him and, obviously, she was working hard on her figure. However, I didn't think her body had a thing to do with his libido. She sat with a sigh of exhaustion.

"We did your eye-gazing exercise. It didn't make us feel more connected if that was your goal. I felt irritated."

She was a midlevel television producer and was used to being frank. I appreciated this quality about her as it somehow invited the same in me.

"I was more curious to see what would come up if there were no distractions—and no words."

"OK, well, I was overwhelmed with disappointment. I felt a wish for a more romantic man. I felt angry he can't be that. He can't even plan a date night."

"Why don't you set it up?"

"I want him to break it."

She was tired of being the leader. If he needed passion, that would be on him to figure out.

"He's always been the more sentimental one. I'm like the guy in so many ways. I'm less emotional, more sexual."

"Imagine you were the underdog. What would that be like?"

"Oh, no way. I've been there before. Insecure, worrying if he was cheating on me, where he was, being the one who was more in love."

That wasn't the interpretation of underdog I expected. To her it meant a lack of safety.

"And he loves you more?"

"He did in the beginning. Now, he's losing interest."

"When's the last time you pined for him, felt your own wanting?"

"Years ago. With my last boyfriend."

"Then why do you initiate sex so much?"

"I want to know he still wants me."

Validation. It's one of the unsexiest reasons to have sex. It's purely egocentric and it's easy to smell. I wonder if this played a role in turning him off. She was content to conquer him each night, without feeling. To her, vulnerability was a fool's endeavor.

"If you don't allow yourself to want, there will be no passion. And he is left alone looking for that kind of connection."

"And I'm withholding."

"Passion requires vulnerability. You can't be top dog."

Why were validation and safety so important to her? I needed to spend time digging around in Tara's personal history, which she wasn't inclined to share. In fact, she didn't want me analyzing her or discussing her past. She reminded me that she wasn't the one who'd signed up for therapy. I wanted to understand why she was guarded, yet so sexual. She wanted a very intimate act, yet was somehow closed off. She eventually shared that she had felt competitive with her mother for her father's affection and had emerged the victor. Her father would take her out on "dates" to work events, even bars when she was a teenager and leave her mother, who had a social phobia, at home. To avenge herself, her mother flirted with Tara's boyfriends and wore provocative clothing in front of them. I wondered if Tara was using sex to win. She loved to feel wanted, to present her body and watch a man's desire.

Mark came in alone for the next session because Tara was on a set in New Orleans. He lumbered in, markedly slower in pace than she, leaned far into my sofa, slacker-style, with his shoulders slumped, legs open, face unshaven. I thought, *Yeah, I can see why she can't surrender to that*. Why couldn't he see it?

I'd briefly worked at an inpatient rehab center for people with drug and alcohol addictions, and Mark reminded me of the experience I had sitting with the clients there. It was as if their souls had been siphoned out; what on the surface appeared to be bright, creative people were instead insubstantial copies of their former selves, listless wraiths. They were hungry, but wanting from a place of emptiness—rather than fullness. I'd often felt drained at the end of my day, a sensation I rarely experience working with sex and relationship issues.

One of my male clients captured it best when he described how he'd felt empty after a one-night stand. He didn't allow that night to matter. He didn't allow the woman to matter. He was trying so hard to keep it impersonal that he ruined the magic. I told him to try another perspective, to have a *petit amour*, a "little love," that just one hour—even a good carnal fuck—with a woman can be imbued with love. Nothing is more existentially dreadful than empty touch.

I know some people are probably reading this thinking, *I've had some really hot, anonymous, matter-less sex*. And, yes, I believe that you're out there having a good time instead of sitting on my couch. But if passion is to be sustainable, sex should matter.

I've learned in practice that eroticism is not always the solution to low libido. Eroticism is titillation. Chemistry is biological. But passion is emotional; its building blocks are expression, openness, longing, an engaged presence, and adoration. It's not the moves, it's the music.

"Did you try the eye-gazing assignment?"

"Yes. It was interesting. I found myself kind of numb. As if she were no different than a chair.

"I'm afraid I married the wrong woman. I keep suggesting that she change something. I asked her to get a tattoo or a piercing. I asked her to dye her hair. She dyed her hair but said she was too old for a tattoo and a piercing. She told me to grow up and to cut down on the porn." He chuckled. "She's right. I feel like no matter how I dress her up—my soul wants something it isn't getting. How do you tell a woman that?"

"So, you learned that if you stop trying to change her, and just look in her eyes and meet who she is...you realize you don't feel love."

"Maybe it's not her fault. I've stopped caring about a lot of things."

"What inspired you before?"

"Telling stories about the good in human nature, resilience, coming together in the face of tragedy. Stories about hope. I felt so alive while writing."

"How long have you had writer's block?"

"Since a bad review came out of my last book. I think I took it to mean that nobody cared about what I had to say. That my words, my thoughts, my whole inner being was deemed uninteresting. My voice just shut down."

"You have to grieve this wound so that you can care about things again. Your wife must matter. Your son. Your own feelings and thoughts. Passion requires the gaze of a poet, to see the beauty in the other. If you want to feel again, look at your wife with curiosity and interest. Passion requires the prurience of an erotic storyteller."

Mark was projecting. Demanding that she be excited—when he couldn't muster it either. Besides, Tara had her own psychological detritus blocking their connection. In the bedroom, both were experiencing the truth of human separateness. As they came together, they were unable to merge. Yet, I wasn't so sure this was as terrible as Mark made it out to be. Two people are rarely in the same perceptual place at the same time. The belief system of Tantra, that through sexual meditations two people can overcome their inherent separateness and become One, with spirit or with each other, seemed a far-fetched idea for these two. I couldn't see them sitting in each other's lap, eye to eye, breathing in rhythm, hands on each other's genitals and hearts.

The Women on My Couch

I don't identify as a practitioner of Tantra or Taoism or anything else. I tossed what I didn't like and culled the best of each. Having this knowledge, I realized that I could get my clients out of the passive, reactive position and into a creative space. If they thought something was degrading or offensive, they would have a new way to reframe it or another direction to lead it. But sometimes my homework inspired by the spiritual traditions—all designed to foster presence and connection—eliminated the distractions that held them together, and they realized their dislike, disgust, numbness, or anger. I think these reactions can be useful. Numbness is an indicator of repression, so we spent some time exploring what Mark truly felt. He was hurt and demoralized as a writer, and angry that Tara didn't understand his pain. She wasn't curious or supportive, and he began to hate her. I asked him what would happen if he shared this with her in words…or expressed his anger sexually.

Mark took what I said to heart. He told me that later the same evening, he was cleaning the kitchen when she came in and carped about the way the dishes were arranged in the dishwasher. Mark swung around from the sink, pushed her up against the wall, pinned her wrists above her head, and said, "You need to be handled properly. I'm going to have to show you who's boss." She let out a smile. He brushed her cheek gently with his finger. Then walked away. He went to his office. Later that night, he walked into the bedroom and found her waiting, wearing lingerie.

One of my favorite things about the *Kama Sutra* is its recognition of the role of aggression in eroticism. In fact, it contains a whole chapter on biting and slapping. Men were warned that women needed to be satisfied lest they become cheerless and prone to fits of epilepsy. And without satisfaction, a woman would lose respect for her man.

As I mentioned, it's a tall order to expect a therapist to help a couple spontaneously feel anything. But Tantra took on that task and so did Taoism and the courtesan Cora Pearl and the poetess Cheeky Minx. The *Kama Sutra* sent people to school for it. They learned how to cause the "opening of the vagina." For example, one passage admonishes, "In order to seduce a woman, it is necessary to know erotic technique. The penis should not be introduced without preparation." The goal was to withhold actual intercourse until she's begging for it.

Tara called the next day and asked if she could come in alone. She wanted to give me her version of that evening. She sounded stressed and impatient on the phone and asked for an appointment immediately. I told her yes and went in an hour early, without my morning coffee. I was a bit under caffeinated when met with her intensity.

"He doesn't want to have sex with me. That fucking hurts enough. I put myself out there, I put on some music, some lingerie, and waited for him in the bedroom. He said he was tired. I freaked out on him."

I asked her to take a breath and slow down, assuming this was the end of her drama. I've seen so many women take it personally when a man suffers low libido. Some even become cruel, putting down his masculinity or sexuality altogether. Tara continued:

"Then, I figured if he can't get into a sexy woman is laying on his bed, then he must be looking at too much porn. So, I went into his office and looked at the browser history on his computer, and right there, I saw where he's getting off. He visits a webcam site. That's real live women on the screen talking to him, doing whatever he tells them. It's cheating! I confronted him and he says it's not cheating. What do you think?"

This was a tough one. Lots of my male clients visit webcam sites. They don't consider it cheating because the woman isn't touchable. She might be real, but so are the girls on screen, so what's the harm in actually asking them to do what you like? To him, this was about his personal and private masturbation experience—not a relational one. Technology makes it difficult to know where the infidelity line is crossed. I define cheating as the betrayal of a negotiated boundary. And depending on the couple, I've seen a wide range of what constitutes infidelity. But in negotiations who preemptively thinks of bringing up webcams?

"When he was in the shower, I took his cell phone and I started to go through it to see if he had any text messages from women. There was nothing. As I was looking through his numbers, I saw the name of one of his college friends. A guy named Ian. I've seen pictures of him on Facebook and he's hot. I sent him a text, from Mark's phone, that said 'Hey, want to get a drink tonight at the Thirsty Crow?'"

"He texted back. 'Yes.'"

I braced myself.

"I walked in and Ian was sitting at the bar, and I walked up and sat down next to him. I said hello and acted like I knew him. He was confused, and I made up a story that I'd met him at a party last year and that we we're both drunk and we flirted. I made up a name and a fake identity. He kept looking around and said he was waiting for someone and I kept ordering us drinks. Eventually, he forgot about Mark and we started kissing. Then, I went to the bathroom, and as I was walking out, I saw Mark come in the front door. Ian saw him and stood up, they hugged. Ian must have texted him to find out where he was. I ran out the back door. Mark came home later. He figured out exactly what I'd done."

"What were you trying to do?"

She started crying. "I want somebody to want me again. That was so stupid. I didn't think it through. Of course, I was going to get caught. I suppose I wanted to, I wanted Mark to see that someone wanted me." She reached down and grabbed my box of tissues and continued to think. "To show him what it feels like to get cheated on, since he wouldn't validate how I felt about the webcam."

"So, do you feel even now?"

"Weirdly, yes, I think guilt feels better than feeling betrayed."

"Is it less vulnerable?"

"Yes, now I'm the villain instead of the victim."

"And still the top dog."

"I guess, but you know, he didn't even seem to care that much. He didn't get outraged. Who doesn't get angry when their wife attempts to cheat?"

"You guys are going about finding passion in all the wrong ways."

"I don't want to do all that stuff, the meditations or role-plays or erotica. Every time I think about that, I feel like something is wrong with me. Your prescriptions remind me that I don't feel passion on my own, that I need help with it. It shouldn't be that hard. A part of me wants to start over. To go to a bar, see a hot guy, flirt, and go home with him."

She seemed resigned. I felt her closing down on me, slipping away. I continued to try to engage her.

"I get it, but play that tape out. Where can it go over time? Maybe you'll end up right back here a few months down the line. Don't you want it to be sustainable?"

"I don't want to put in the effort…with Mark."

I was disappointed. I had hope, as I always do, that our work together would help them find what they were looking for. But with Mark and Tara, I was running into the limits of what I had to offer. Learning the skills of loving or seduction doesn't necessarily work when two people don't like each other. There was a glimmer of hope that night he stood up to her, but the buildup of ordinary resentments rested in his bones. Remaining open hearted and ready to surrender is an ideal that's hard to attain in the context of a real relationship.

Psychology has helped me understand the barriers to feeling passion. So much gets in the way: our parents, our past, our culture. I have to field defense mechanisms, personality traits, and transference like constant missiles exploding on my Pollyanna front. In reality, to get to the ascendant place of love and lust, people have to work for it. Neither Mark nor Tara wanted to do that. They both took the easy way out: him, porn and drink; her, work and child.

In many of my couples therapy cases, couples are successful in overcoming the rancor and finding Eros again. And others just want to blow it all up and start over.

Amber

Guys had tried before. Amber would sweep away their probing hands or grab their shoulders and pull them up if they tried to go down on her. Then, one night after a party, her boyfriend Dave picked her up, slung her over his shoulder, carried her to his bedroom, laid her upon his bed, tied her hands to the post, and went down on her. After forty-five minutes, and shooting pain in his jaw, he gave up. Amber came to see me, not of her own accord, but at his request.

It's not ideal when a client comes to therapy at the behest of someone else; they tend to be half-hearted about change, and some even rebel against the therapist. I began by asking for her perspective on what happens in the bedroom.

"It's like I'm on stage, with my legs spread open, forced to reveal the most ugly part of my body to an audience that I really want to impress."

Amber's words were dramatic, yet clearly articulated the subtle shame and vulnerability many women experience when sharing their nudity. In my practice, I've never heard a guy speak about his body this way.

She continued,

"Vaginas. Let's face it. They're not attractive. They're wet and oozy, they bleed, they have these weird flaps. There's no way you're going to sell me that my pussy is a Goddess or any of that bullshit. I even hate the word 'pussy.' I hate the word 'vagina,' too. I just prefer to keep it tucked into my jeans," she said with a wry grin.

"And Dave is right there, up close, trying to show it some love."

"Ugh, it was so terrible. He was working so hard down there, and I knew it wasn't going anywhere. What a fucking chore. Why aren't orgasms easier?"

She had a good point: orgasms aren't easy. They require focus, and it's easy to get distracted. Yet, she didn't come across as concerned. She wanted a laugh, a chuckle, a grin…anything but my earnest inquiry. I purposely deprived her and held a serious demeanor.

"Maybe he likes your vagina."

"God, you said 'vagina.' What else can we call it? I hate when women make up cutesy names like hoo-ha or cooch. Let's just call it 'down there.' I don't know why guys like what they like. Breasts. They're obsessed with those, too. I have no idea why—they're freak-in' udders."

"And can he touch your breasts?"

"Yeah, he can fondle my udders." She laughed.

Amber identified herself as a filmmaker. She'd never worked on a movie but had done a few "shorts" in film school. She was also a comedian, a dog-walker, an unpaid studio intern and was contemplating law school as a backup plan. She lived in Sherman Oaks, a neighborhood on the back side of the Hollywood Hills. For some reason I still don't understand, it's been deemed uncool.

Amber was candid, yet hostile. Her frank answers were not honest attempts to connect with me. I continued trying to engage her with open-ended questions.

"What did you learn about your body growing up?"

"Hah. Really? Well, I guess I shouldn't be surprised; you're a therapist. Let's see, God, you're really going after it right away. I don't even know if I like you yet."

"OK, now I feel like I'm on stage. Like you're auditioning me, and, yes, I hope you will like me," I said.

"Is that some kind of reverse psychology?"

"No, it's my honest response. Seems like you're trying to figure out if I'm safe."

"A lot of therapists are fucked up themselves."

"Sure, we're people. Look, if it takes some time for you to trust me, I'm willing to be patient."

"Thanks, I have that 'on stage' feeling right now—it's something about you. I don't feel totally comfortable."

I had to stop and wonder if it was me. Was I too clinical? My professional responses too rehearsed? Perhaps I viewed her as a case—not a person. Maybe I should have laughed at her jokes or told a few myself.

"I'm glad you're letting me know how you're reacting to me. I'm willing to consider it's me, if you're willing to look at yourself, too."

"I guess I have that same 'on stage' feeling as if you're examining my ugly parts."

"And what do you imagine I think of you?"

She sat quiet for a moment and shed a tear.

"I'm getting nervous."

"Take a breath with me."

"Oh, Lord, please don't say 'take a breath'—such a therapist-y thing to say."

She sighed, sarcastically loud.

The session was over and I had another client waiting. The moment was lost. Amber's defense was clear. Fight. Fight me, fight my ideas, fight the relief of a simple breath. Why did this young woman have her javelin pointed at me? I had a sense that she wanted to let me in, and that she wanted to let Dave in, that there was a longing to be seen. Nevertheless, she was going to make me work to get close to her.

I wish I could say that Amber's disdain for her vagina was rare, that she had some diagnosable disorder, like body dysmorphia. But I've had tons of similar cases—even millennials who are loathing their vaginas and shunning orgasms when guys are offering. This aversion runs deep in our consciousness, challenges our liberal ideals, and shows up in the bravest of women.

Collectively, women are still in recovery (if not still actively being repressed by religions or governments in some parts of the world). Body shaming has a long history, but so does body reverence. In fact, humanity has undergone a total reversal from the ancient past, when sex and earth and woman were erotic and divine—like, together, at the same time. There was Shaivism in ancient India, Goddess-worshipping civilizations in Europe, the bawdy pre-Roman Etruscans, and Native American tribes that celebrated the human body. In fact, there are so many examples, to discuss them all is beyond the scope of this book. I will tell the story here of the culture that was the most profound for me. What was meant to be an innocuous visit to a museum on a Sunday afternoon ended up leading me to Greece and to a discovery that forever changed the way I viewed my body.

I'd read in the *L.A. Times* about a new museum exhibit at the Getty Villa in Malibu dedicated to Aphrodite. Finally, I would find her. I would come face to face with an original Goddess of love, beauty, and all erotic pleasures. I barely allowed myself to breathe as I made my way to the museum. Aphrodite would no longer be a figure of my imagination, an abstract source of inspiration. The idea of her was rife with my projections. She was a yearning in my soul for a celebration of women's desire, an affirmation of our true nature. I'd been long weary of the way women were portrayed in modern media, for in all the sexed-up imagery, my lust is rarely evoked—only self-consciousness—creating an insidious molding of identity, an internal sculpture. Images do that; they change us. They have the power to tell us who we are in the world. What would this Aphrodite statue mirror back to me? How would I see myself in her presence?

I drove along the coastal highway, and perched up in the hills was the museum. The building is a replica of an ancient Roman villa, with elaborate gardens, fountains, a pool, and pomegranate trees—all overlooking the ocean. A proper setting for this meeting. I decided to attend a lecture on Aphrodite by a classics professor to learn all I could.

I arrived early to browse the artwork on the many jugs, reliefs, sculptures, mirrors, and other artifacts. There are two themes in Greek art: fighting and fucking. The Aphrodite exhibit was dedicated solely to the latter. There was group sex, oral sex, magical creature sex, and even a man penetrating a goat surrounded by satyrs (those randy half-man, half-goat creatures with giant erect penises that always look menacingly upon their prey).

Then, there she was, standing in the center of the exhibit. Tall, marble, blank faced. I paused in reverence. She seemed vacant. There was no stirring inside of me. I stood there, only aware of what I wanted from her, not an idol to worship but a reminder that a woman's lust was bestowed by the gods, that we had a divine blessing to revel in our lush sensuality. However, my interpretation was not what the Greeks intended. I didn't know much about Greek civilization, so in the lecture, I was eager to learn about the meaning of these images and this culture that seemed to be so blatantly sexual.

The first fact that struck me was that the Greeks weren't into love. Now, those already studied in ancient Greek culture won't be as surprised to learn that when Aphrodite and her winged cohort Eros bestowed love upon their human subjects, the humans weren't so grateful. The spark of romance that we require today to feel turned on was not a welcomed part of Greek sexuality. Love and desire were seen as afflictions, kinds of maladies. I wrote down one of their aphorisms in my notebook:

"You should flee Eros."

—Archaism

With no celebration of love, I already wasn't jiving with the Greeks when the lecturer dealt the second blow. I had asked specifically about the Greek perspective on women's sexual desire, and she replied, "Good Greek wives should not feel desire for their husbands. These feelings are for men." She further explained that in Greek society, women were not a part of the social, economic, and political spheres at all.

I couldn't grasp that a culture would have a female love and sex *Goddess*, with shrines and tons of art depicting women in scenes of erotic abandon, yet this was only for men. I waited until the lecture was over to ask more questions.

"Look at that jug," I said to the professor, trying to make my case for what appeared obvious. "Those women look pretty sensual to me. There has to be more to the story of their erotic lives."

"Eros wasn't for women," she replied.

Her response seemed like some weird, absolutist generalization. How can an entire gender be labeled as nonsexual?

"The women depicted in this art are slaves and courtesans, not everyday women. In fact, everyday women would have never seen this art," she explained. She said that the art was for those hedonistic man parties, the famed symposiums.

I was still confused by the images in the art of women looking gratified. I saw a mirror that featured a woman having sex with a man. She was reaching her head back to kiss him and a little winged Eros was flying over them with a victory flag. Surely, this must be evidence of female satisfaction. I pointed and asked, "Why are there so many images like this on women's perfume bottles and mirrors?"

"Aphrodite helped women to inspire desire in men, not to feel it for themselves."

"You've got to have some example of art or literature that is solely about women's Eros for me," I said. I wasn't letting go, and she started to look annoyed.

"Nothing," she replied. "Well, there is one poet, named Sappho, but there are only fragments."

Then the professor excused herself. She'd had enough of my inquisition. I'd come to the museum seeking historical support for my hypothesis that women are just as sexual as men, that women's sensuality was celebrated, and that Aphrodite would be proof. I left with more questions than answers. I decided that I didn't get the whole story, that I'd gotten a one-sided tale told by those who paid for and created the art on display at the museum. But why didn't the professor know about other sources of information? She had dedicated her career to Aphrodite and all she could give me was one poet?

I went to the museum bookstore, bought books, and then went home. I strolled into a coffee shop in my neighborhood, new books under my arm, and sat down. A nearby woman asked, "What's that you're reading?" I told her the story about my experience at the museum. I explained that I was looking for answers and my frustration that "there must be more to the story…"

The woman replied, "There is."

She was an art historian who specialized in female representations in art. She told me that there were resistance movements in the Greek empire and secretive cults that supported female sexuality. If I wanted to get the most important story about sex in the ancient Western world, I needed to learn about the civilization that preceded the Greeks—the Minoans. I recalled the name from my college world history course and that was about it. So, I bought more books.

The Minoans were based on the island of Crete. They built one of the earliest advanced states in the Mediterranean and were a successful economic power in the region. Most importantly for our purposes, the Minoans produced extraordinary art depicting women in a manner unseen in later generations.

To see the Minoan artifacts, one must go the island of Crete, where the Minoans settled as early as 7000 BC in a town we now call Knossos. I really wanted to understand what life was like *before* women's sexuality went underground, so I decided to go to Crete.

Amber came back for her second session. As she walked past my desk and took a seat, I noticed how tiny she was, her childlike frame, short and thin, in contrast to her linebacker presence. Her black hair was cut into an old-school bowl cut, straight and equal length all the way around, and she wore large, red eyeglasses and a plain green T-shirt with brown corduroy pants. She placed her leather bag on the floor next to my sofa, and I could see a book slipping out. Ugh, it was Henry Miller's *Tropic of Cancer*. I wished I could prescribe her a little D. H. Lawrence instead.

"Alright, doc, I'm ready for this. I've got my game face on. Let's talk oral sex." She laughed.

"Why do you think he wants to do that?" I began.

"Cuz, that's what guys want."

"Why?"

"Cuz, they're guys."

"So, they're doing it for themselves?"

"Yes, I have no idea why they get turned on by the things that they do."

"What if he wants to share something with you, express love, worship your body?"

"Worship? Are you gonna get New Age on me?"

"Could you allow that?"

"I'd want to make fun of it."

I was getting tired of the court jester act.

"That would elicit your contempt? Someone wanting to adore your body?"

She paused.

"This is reverence. For you. And you want to bat it down with sarcasm. Help me understand that."

"Most of the guys I've hooked up with are in and out, they don't care if I finish, and to be honest, I'm more comfortable with that. I see sex for what it is, a crude and swift act. It doesn't mean anything to them, so why should it mean something to me?" She held my gaze, as if challenging me.

"Do you think Dave wants it to mean something?"

"I guess."

"OK, no jokes here. Can you allow that for yourself?"

"I want to. I do. I want to let it in."

She was all pluck and spirit, but where was her sense of entitlement? Belief that her body was significant? That pleasure was important? Why wasn't this instilled in her? These questions are hard to answer without examining the environment a woman is raised in, so we drew up a genogram, a family map that included the entire extended family, grandparents, even great-grandparents. The drawing looked like a tree and visually provided the big picture. We charted her family relationships: who was close or distant, who was violent, who was sick or addicted, and it was a powerful moment to see the generational patterns laid out before her eyes—a moment of realizing her emotional legacy.

"I grew up in an Evangelical Christian household, so we never talked about sex except to say that there's no sex before marriage. Church isn't protecting the sanctity of sex; they're making people feel ashamed of it. I don't recall ever learning to feel proud of my body."

"What about your mom? Did she seem to feel comfortable with sexuality?"

"Are you kidding? No way."

"And her mom?"

"Grandma?" Laughs. "I have no idea. She was married to a minister."

"Let's consider what lessons the women in your family learned about their bodies—not just sexually, but in general."

"They're from rural Appalachian Mountains. Generations of factory workers and miners originally from Wales and Scotland. They worked hard and they played hard. A bunch of them are alcoholics, my mom's two sisters were molested by my granddad. One of them never married; she moved to California, and the other is super-religious. My mom was spared because my grandma divorced him and moved away with the girls."

"Any other abuse in the family?"

"They're all violent sometimes," her voice hardened. "My uncle slaps my aunt, she slaps the kids, those kids used to hit us, my mom hit my dad, he hit her back a few times."

"And has anybody hurt you?"

"Of course, but that was a long time ago....

My mom used to hit me, call me useless, waste of money and space. She was a single mom, and she felt the pressure of money all the time, and we were a burden to her. She made us work in the house instead of doing homework."

"Sounds like you felt exploited."

She started to stare off into space, so I halted my questioning. There were tears in her eyes, the first sign of softness. I felt a swell of kindness toward her.

"I appreciate you sharing this with me. You're safe right now, right here in this room."

"Why bring all this up? What's it going to do for me?" Her questions continued to challenge me, but finally she was rolling over, showing me her belly.

"Is it hard to remember or to tell me?"

"Both. I feel sad to think of it. The whole cycle of people taking life out on each other. Love letting everybody down."

"Hard to trust people. Hard to trust even me?" I asked.

"Yes. But I can see that you want to care. I can see that Dave cares, but somehow what you're offering seems unreal, something strange that I can't process, like I'm helplessly there unable to take it."

Amber never learned how to receive love. The bodies of her ancestors had been exploited as workers, and they had passed around their anger like a hot potato. The only relief came from alcohol or Christian revival. The deep roots of bodily disregard were part of a larger cultural history. The women of her past were immigrants: poor, hard workers. Some were molested, some were abused, some self-destructed, and others sought refuge in piety. This told me a lot about why Amber hates the word "vagina."

Amber wanted to escape Appalachia, and she was the first person in her entire extended family to go to college. However, neither the distance nor the education could heal her wound. Oral sex brought up unconscious barriers to sharing a vulnerable, naked self. Her relationship with David was a shot at a healthy relationship. She'd met him at a comedy improv class. He was Jewish, came from a loving family, and everything he had to offer—his erudition, his warmth, his urbanity—she wanted to receive and to become, even though it felt foreign and made her roil with insecurity.

I arrived on the Greek island of Crete eager to find what the art historian from the coffee shop wanted me to discover. The first written language of the Minoans hasn't been deciphered, so the iconography left on the walls and artifacts would be my only information. The Minoans have inspired controversy and fantasy, so I had to be cautious about drawing conclusions based on my wishes. Fortunately, I brought my husband with me, a man serious about academic rigor. He carried along archeological journals and textbooks, functioning like a crossing guard ready to blow the whistle if I moved toward any errant generalizations. I was enthusiastic about the rare opportunity to view images unbound from any definitive narrative. I would have to learn through the raw, nonverbal communication of the image and my own sentience; such a perfect way to learn about an erotic world. I sat with each image, breathed it in, and waited for impressions to register.

At the museum, I didn't find any sex. I saw a grand total of two images of a man and woman holding hands and looking at each other. I was thinking, *Where's the sex? Why did she send me here?*

What I did see were breasts. Topless women. Everywhere. On wall art, on pottery, on engraved gold seal stones. This culture would have been surrounded in its architecture and daily life with pictures of bare-chested women. I decided to switch my focus to the meaning of this breast extravaganza. The sheer ubiquity of them and the curious way the bosom was displayed must've had an important story to tell.

The standard outfit worn by the Minoan woman was a long, flowing skirt, full of color and designs such as flowers and geometric lines. She would have a corset around her waist that laced up and then stopped just below the bust, lifting it up and out. A small, open cardigan that covered the back, shoulders, and upper arms topped off the ensemble. Basically, the entire body was covered except for the chest. It was as if the purpose of the clothing was to frame and present the breasts.

In most of the art, the breasts are large, prominent. With all the pomp of the attire, I wasn't under the impression that this display meant breasts were un-self-conscious body parts (like those of a French woman I once saw sitting topless on the beach eating a sandwich and crocheting a scarf). The intentional uplifting and presenting implied some significance. What that meaning was nobody knows. But as I sat contemplating my experience of the female figures before me, I realized that this portrayal didn't fit into my perceptual history of breasts.

The programming of my gaze was to view the breasts as sexy, but the Minoan artworks didn't appear to be constructed with the intention of sexual allure—believe me, that's what I wanted to read into it. Further, the images didn't seem maternal either. There were almost no representations of pregnancy, breastfeeding, or interaction with children. I was confused. So, if the bosom wasn't sexual or maternal, then what was it? They certainly didn't go bare-breasted due to a lack of clothing. There was no indication they were prostitutes, courtesans, or slaves. In fact, the actions these ladies were performing while topless indicated something else.

One of my favorites was a gold impression of a skirted, topless woman standing on a mountaintop, holding forth a scepter, flanked by lions, with a male adorant at the base of the mountain. I was excited by the image, but it didn't resonate with any experience I'd had myself. It seemed unreal, like a comic character. Charges of forgery and deceit had been leveled against this image until similar ones were excavated at different times in other locations.

Then, there was the infamous "snake Goddess," a figurine found at every souvenir shop on the island. It's a woman with her arms wide open, a snake writhing in each hand, flowers in her hair, and a cat atop her head. Her breasts are plunging forward, erect, implying the same formidable effect of an erect phallus. The woman has a bold look about her face, making direct eye contact. I had never seen a breast evoke such audacity, respect, and awe.

After viewing this statuette in the museum, I went to a souvenir shop to buy one to keep by my computer while writing this chapter. I picked out a four-inch figurine, and the proprietress, a stout elder Greek woman, forcefully told me, "No!" and picked up the largest version, about the size of my arm. "This is the good one," she declared. I was afraid to contest. And my poor husband lugged the heavy statue the rest of our trip. When his bag went through the x-ray in U.S. Customs, the security agent asked him to explain the strange outline of a woman with a giant bosom that appeared on the monitor. "Is that an angel?" the agent asked. "No...can't be," he pondered. A small crowd of curious male TSA agents gathered.

"Uh, it's a Goddess," my husband tepidly replied.

"But she's holding snakes in her hands," the agent said.

"It's a *snake* Goddess, man."

"Um, we're going to have to take this out and have a look."

They all snickered, and then let him pass on through.

Clearly, culture impacts the way women view their body: its worth, its function, its beauty or non-beauty. It's all relative. I wished that Amber could see her vagina the way I had seen the Minoan breasts. I wasn't sure how to carry the experience back to my clients.

Amber had decided that she wanted to think about her body in a different way. But she didn't know how to make the change. And she had a good point. How does one make a radical change in perspective? One look at her family tree showed how hard it can be. She would be the first woman to break the repetition. But without any model or guidance, how would she create the change?

We agreed that she wouldn't push herself to receive oral sex, that she could wait until she truly felt she was ready to share her body and sexuality from a place of pride. David had been very patient and supportive. In the meantime, she agreed to give him oral sex, which didn't bring her any anxiety. I knew our process would take time, and the following is only a small window into what happened in therapy.

Amber wanted to try on hats before making a decision about who, sexually, she wanted to become. So, she decided to sign up for yoga, meditation, and pole dancing to start (all her ideas). Over the course of a few weeks, she took classes and kept a journal of her reactions to share with me.

"Yoga was boring. I don't get why all my friends are into it. Meditation was even more boring, but the instructor was cute, so I went back."

I wasn't surprised by her reaction to slowing down. Amber was used to being amped all the time, so sitting on the floor with no mental stimulation and trying to pay attention to her body for the first time must have felt like watching a clock tick. I encouraged her to stay with it, to access that well-being and sexual energy that comes with relaxation. Amber decided she preferred a more active approach. She wanted to feel like she was doing —rather than being.

"I went to a pole dance class with my best friend and it was really fun. The class was taught by a gay guy who wore cut-off jeans shorts and red sequined high heels. Awesome."

Amber went to several classes, rehearsed the routine, and then bought some little shorts and heels and decided she would surprise David. After dinner and a couple of cocktails, she sat David down and told him to wait while she went in the bedroom and changed into her outfit. Then, she came out into her living room and performed the routine she'd learned in class.

"He loved it, and I think he was truly shocked."

"How was it for you?"

"Fun. I pulled off the routine really well, but I didn't feel turned on. When we went to have sex after, I wasn't wet."

"Where was your mind?"

"Aware that I was being watched."

Amber had put herself back up on stage—separate and above the audience, where she can make jokes or do a dance or act out an emotional expression as she does in her films, all from a distance. Getting down on the same level with her audience, to have an interaction instead of a presentation, brought out her insecurity, both in the therapy room and in the bedroom.

"Did you feel any sexual desire when you danced?"

"No. If all I do is learn how to shake my ass like Beyoncé, then I'm still missing something."

I was glad that they both had fun, and that dance classes helped Amber to enjoy her body rather than disparage it, but she remained an out-of-body observer. Dance can be a tool for connecting to one's body or sexuality; however, it's most powerful as an emotional expression rather than as empty, stereotyped movements.

Behavior follows reinforcement. Because sexiness is a commodity in modern society, bodies and commercialism are weaved together. Identities become mottled by what pop stars, advertisers, movie stars, or Twitter influencers tell us is cool. Ordinary people play back those dictates, using the same sexual postures to sell themselves or their businesses online. It's a sociosexual feedback loop, an exchange of ideas on social status—not real lust. The cost to the average woman is an external-ized sexuality that lacks intrinsic motivation and spontaneity. In fact, the more exposure women have to hypersexual media, the more self-conscious and the *less sexual* they feel. Even Amber, an unconventional, thoughtful young woman, rejected searching inward for her sexuality. I wanted to show her a different image. I pulled out my snake Goddess statue and set it before her.

"Oh, my God," she furrowed her brow and moved in closer.

"What do you feel when you look at this?" I asked, hoping this could be the moment I wanted it to be.

Her eyes opened wide. I wasn't sure if she was coming up with some witty rejoinder or really considering the statue before her.

"I don't know…I'm kinda scared of her…intimidated. Oh, oh, I get it. She is exposed, yet fierce—this is something I want. I fucking want that."

"You can have it. You can be the first woman in your family to own your body this way."

She began to cry, and my eyes filled with tears, and we sat silent for a moment.

"Are you gonna, like, pull out some snakes now?"

"No." I laughed. "Can we take this opportunity to have some empa-thy for everything your body has been through?"

"OK."

"Just close your eyes and take a breath. Let's face the truth. You've been exploited and abused. Let's just pause on that truth for a moment. Remembering what that has felt like…"

She sat silent.

"Place your hand where you feel it."

She placed her hand over her heart.

"Let's surround that feeling with tenderness."

A single tear fell down her cheek.

"Silently repeat after me. I'm sorry I've ignored you. I'm sorry I've turned against you, too."

Her lips quivered as she began to cry.

"Repeat after me. I'm here for you now. I will give you the respect you deserve."

We had to repeat this inner dialogue over the course of several weeks. She wasn't going to make peace with her family, but she could make peace with her body. I could have directed her toward systems of belief like Taoism or Tantra that offer a path toward viewing the body as divine, but she didn't want anything to do with spirituality. She'd been too hurt by Christianity. I used poetry, art, and writings that affirmed her body. Amber also spent time at home in front of a mirror gazing at her body, fighting through thoughts that it's ugly, staring with a forced compassion until she cried, then breathing, and, with all the courage she could muster, saying, "I honor you."

A few months later, she'd opened her legs, and her soul, for David.

Reflecting upon the Minoans, I contemplated my own body. One specific memory was about the summer before I entered high school, when I'd overheard a neighbor boy, an early crush, tell a friend that boys wouldn't like me until I "gained some weight and grew some boobs." Terrified of rejection, I commenced drinking milkshakes every night. An immediate emotional imprint had occurred: I *felt* small chested. I felt smaller, less significant. The social learning was that size matters and that my chest would be scrutinized by others. This ongoing messaging throughout my adolescence disconnected me from my breasts, which became alien, numb, disembodied.

The American relationship with breasts can be summarized in one word: weird. Women are fraught with self-consciousness about size or firmness, what to reveal, what not to reveal. Some women invest in implants, yet any ostentatious display can elicit scorn from other women (i.e., "Her boobs are fake"). When breastfeeding in public places, women are supposed to hide the act, preferably in a restroom.

A look at our language further displays American weirdness. There are words like "melons" and "knockers," which are silly, or words like "rack" and "tits," which are harsh, vulgar even. Then there's the word "boob," which also means idiot.

The Women on My Couch

Breasts are an emotionally loaded body part. Contact with mother's breast is our first sexual experience, the first communion with another body. It is the taking in of nourishment, comfort, and love in a pure, uncomplicated form that doesn't exist in adulthood. This simple, life-giving act is of great magnificence: the magic of nature to nurture life. To trivialize the breast reflects an inability to marvel at the universe.

In stark contrast, I realized that this snake Goddess sitting next to my computer, with her great, imposing chest, appeared to be in full possession of her body. The Minoan women, who lived 2,000 years before Christ, danced, corsets off, with their breasts like ripe pears balanced atop small waists and ample, ebullient hips and bottoms. Their curves, drawn in exaggerated, sinuous lines, seemed a celebration of the natural form. The dancers were surrounded by chrysalises, trees, and water, which are features widely accepted by archeologists as demonstrating a spiritual connection with nature. The tone of their worship looked exuberant. There are lots of arms raised, hair flying, and hips swaying to the music of the lyre. These pictures rupture the layers of extraterrestrial meanings later civilizations have attached to the nude body: morals, beauty ideals, egotism, commercialized manipulations.

Yet the Minoans are not to be reduced to some ancient hippie utopian culture. In fact, this civilization has been the subject of overzealous reconstruction since the swashbuckling British explorer Sir Arthur Evans put his money into the excavation process. He took the liberty of finishing the fragmented frescoes himself, which almost discredited him and the story of the Minoan women right along with it. The guy actually hired painters to re-paint entire women based on a few fragments of hair or jewelry . In the world of archeology, that's outrageous. Yet, that's how it stands today, and tourists visit by the millions. The night before my trip to the infamous ruins of Knossos on Crete, I'd asked fellow travelers for their opinions on the enhanced frescoes. People had either unquestionably embraced a peaceful mother Goddess culture or had dismissed it all as imagination.

Fortunately, I'd recently learned of an exciting new development—the discovery of an ancient town on the island of Santorini that had been preserved by a volcanic eruption. I decided to go look for the intact wall paintings of the famous Minoan women. There, on an island synonymous with parties and seafood, was an excavation site that should be grabbing the attention of the world. There, I hoped, the controversy over the truth of the Minoans could be resolved, and the truth about women's place in history revealed.

In one of the best tax write-offs of my career, my husband and I sailed to Santorini. When we arrived to the excavation site, called Akrotiri, we discovered that all of the art was gone. There was nothing but stone and dirt. I asked an attendant, "Where is the art?"

"Not on view," he said. "It's been removed and is under restoration. You can see two pieces at the museum in town, but they're about to close."

I was crestfallen. We'd have to wait for a bus to get us back to town. There was no way we'd make it in time. I looked at my husband and said, "Noooooooo!"

My husband, Francis, who was also caught up in the archeological mysteries, was not about to travel all the way to Santorini and not see one of these wall paintings or deal with my mood. Ever bold, he went out to the street, waived down car after car, and pleaded with the drivers to take us to the museum, telling our story as if our need to view this art was some life-threatening emergency. Finally, a sympathetic woman agreed to take us. We began chatting in the car and found out that she was a tour guide for the actual excavation site, had a degree in archeology, and had photos of the unavailable frescoes in her car!

"I can show you photos of everything that has been uncovered so far."

With the controversy of Arthur Evans in the back of my mind, and my wish that his extravagant and reckless vision was correct, I was blown away by what I saw, an abundance of well-preserved scenes of women in full regalia of their lush ancient glamour. They were all highly stylized with hair adorned with flowers, necklaces, giant hoop earrings, bracelets, eyeliner, rouge, lipstick. Their hair was long and carefully coiffed. And their breasts were in full bloom.

The Women on My Couch

One fresco featured a woman on an elevated throne receiving tribute from a procession of women carrying votives and pots. In other paintings official-looking women presided over various public events. Men were catching fish, harvesting crops, rowing boats, or assuming positions of spiritual supplication. These ladies were clearly leaders in public rituals. And although they were beautiful, they seemed grounded rather than ethereal, solid bodies held upright in proud postures.

The Akrotiri excavations tell us that women held an important status in a society that flourished for 1,500 years before they were demoted by the Greeks. Although I can't say anything definitive about the sexual practices of these exquisitely drawn women, I will say that the ability to feel sexual is inextricably linked to the worth of women's bodies in a sociocultural context. Women appeared to have a high social status, and reverence for the female form was a central part of their culture. This is a pretty powerful message. Just for contrast, consider the role of women under the soon-to-arrive Greeks.

In the Greek empire, women disappeared from public life altogether. They were barred from political and social life. Men and women were socialized to believe that a woman's body was inferior, and the female form was desexualized. It was important for a woman's body to be covered, and the public narrative was that women were not sexual, only men were. Men experienced Eros toward primarily other men, and a woman wasn't to experience desire. She was supposed to seduce by making herself as attractive as possible—though her form was generally viewed as utilitarian.

An example from an actual handbook from the Stoics states:

> The only advantage women have got is to be marriageable, they begin to make themselves smart and set all their hopes on this. We must take pains to make them understand that they are really honored for nothing but a modest and decorous life.
> —*The Manual*, by Epictetus

There, of course, was debate about women, love, and sex—this was Greece after all. Socrates was a proponent of all three, but his was not the prevailing attitude. Most Greek men were interested in the male physical ideal. The young man was their sexual idol. Although Greek men have a reputation for an expansive sexuality, actually they were obsessed with a singular object: the perfect, strong physique. They also had a bunch of prudish rules, such as civilized Greek men were not to show arousal and were not to give oral sex or to be on the receiving end of a penis—for this would distort their beautiful faces or disrespect their ideal bodies. Those positions were only for inferiors: slaves, foreigners, women. Male horniness and arousal were split off and projected onto satyrs and foreigners.

According to Thomas Cahill, author of *Why the Greeks Matter*, the tenor of Greek sexuality was impersonal, exploitive, brutish, narcissistic, and vulgar. Their sexual behavior mirrored their society's prevailing virtues, which were demonstrations of conquest and domination. The Romans, who shared these values, literally took it to the next level of masculinization by dressing up Aphrodite (Venus) in a helmet, arming her with a shield, and expanding her powers to include military success.

This is obviously a dramatic difference from the dancing Minoans—and an important shift in the history of women. How exactly did the change happen? Nobody knows for sure. Akrotiri was destroyed by a massive volcanic eruption, and around the same time a natural disaster, perhaps an earthquake, destroyed civilization on Crete. Marauding pirates seized control of the Aegean Sea, and the last Minoans sought refuge in the mountains.

I contacted Dr. Nanno Marinatos, archeology professor at the University of Illinois and author of a book about the Akrotiri excavations called *Art and Religion in Thera*, and asked her if she thought the discoveries would change the way the West understands its history. "Yes," she said, and that "due to the volcanic preservation, we will have more information than ever about this early period." Dr. Marinatos, privy to excavations not yet made public, includes a series of illustrations in her book to give us a peek at what will hopefully be available to all in the future. She believes that Sir Arthur Evans may indeed have been right all along.

The contrast between the Greeks and the Minoans illustrates that the perception of sexuality can shift. Human sexuality is not static; it changes according to the mores of a culture. Further, sex gets weaved into matters of security, economics, and politics. According to the Greek archeologist Yannis Hamilakis, cultures don't just evolve in one forward direction of progress; they move back and forth and back again.

When I think about the dilemmas of my clients, I've learned to integrate psychology, culture, and history into my understanding, to consider how sexuality mirrors our culture's prevailing virtues. Does she believe her body is attractive, inferior, weak, strong, utilitarian, or sacred? Is desire for him, for her, for both? Does she feel at home on a stage, in a field, or in a bedroom? Is sex transactional, hierarchical, ego-driven, ego-less, part of nature, or covered in latex and slathered with lube, eyes behind a mask? I'm not concerned with right or wrong—but with who makes these decisions.

When I see the unconstrained bosom of the snake Goddess, I see a self-governing woman, one who owns her body and, I imagine, her sexual desire as well. I wonder if the Minoan women felt as mighty in their sexuality as did the woman depicted standing on a mountaintop holding a scepter, if they felt the right to receive an orgasm the way the woman seated on a throne felt the right to receive offerings. I doubt that a Minoan woman worried about the size of her breasts or scrutinized the busts of her sisters as they danced topless under the trees. Given that nipples are featured on everything from vases to religious figurines, I also doubt they were asked to breastfeed in private. I doubt they believed that sexual pleasure and desire and their bodies belonged to the realm of men.

The Minoan paintings surrounded them in public life. The frescoes were not hidden or tucked away, not part of some marginal cult. Images are important to our identities, and I'm hopeful that women like Amber will create new images. I told her, as I tell many of my clients: don't let other people tell the story of who you are. Don't be just a consumer of other people's ideas. What do you want to express, feel, or be? Go forth and put that out in the world—and support other women in their expressions.

As this snake Goddess sitting next to my computer stares at me with all her gravitas, as I complete this chapter, I'm reminded that she is lushly feminine, but not demure or silly or empty. She is powerful. And, if anything else, she reminds me to put my shoulders back, push my chest forward, hold my head high—that alone was worth my journey all the way to Crete.

Postscript

Notes from the Couch

There was a great deal of material that didn't make it into the book, largely because there wasn't room to include everything and still have a story that flows. There were studies and poems and cultural facts that had all shaped me as a clinician and a woman. Discovering the stories, and cultures in this book brought me great joy, so I thought I'd share some bonus material in a diary form rather than let it sit in the dusty files of Microsoft Word where it would never be opened again.

Note:
What happens when women take the lead?
Inspiration from research on speed dating
and lesbian relationships

I like to ask my single clients about what happens when they go out to meet men at a bar. When they see a man they're attracted to—what do they do? I want to know if they approach that person directly or if they send nonverbal signals, like a smile or eye contact.

What do you do with your attraction? Take action, wait, paralyze? I want to know if they walk into a bar *expecting* to choose someone to hook up with or if they tend to wait to be chosen. Even a woman who subtly flirts can still be actively choosing, feeling a sense of entitlement. This active frame of mind may, in fact, have a huge impact on the experience of desire.

The Women on My Couch

Daniel Bergner, in *What Women Want*, a journalistic review of the modern research on desire, ends the book with a study that upends social norms. The scene is a speed dating event. Men and women sit at a long table facing each other, and every few minutes a bell rings. The men get up and move to the next lady. Afterward, both men and women make a list of who they were attracted to. Tallies showed that men were consistently attracted to larger numbers of women than women were to men. This was initially accepted as evidence of men's almost indiscriminate attraction resulting from their need to inseminate and of women's choosier nature.

However, two researchers, Eli Finkel from Northwestern University and Paul Eastwick at the University of Texas, questioned the structure of these big speed dating studies. Finkel and Eastwick decided to set up a speed dating test of their own, this time with one variable adjusted: after the bell rang, the men remained seated. The women got up and moved to the next candidate.

The results were dramatically different.

Now women reported experiencing attraction, as much and as indiscriminately as the men had in previous studies. With one shift in the structure of the experiment, the results were completely turned around. Finkel and Eastwick's redesign casts doubt on the speed dating megastudy results, which seemed so consistent that they must reflect some truth about men and women.

Social structure influences our perception of desire. *As women are taken out of the passive, responding role and asked to become active agents, a shift takes place.*

What happens when we remove the social norms that support the differences we see between men and women? Another answer comes from research on lesbian sexuality. Without men in the scenario, the shape of women's desire is altered—radically. Jane Ussher published a study in the journal *Feminism & Psychology* that reveals "young lesbians' experience of desire can sometimes be positive and powerful, freed from the constraints of the heterosexual matrix." Ussher's study on sex drive provides insight into why some large-scale studies deliver dour news about women's sexual appetites. Ussher's study was much smaller, yet the volunteers revealed greater diversity and fluidity.

Ussher's results are likely due to her unconventional method. Rather than hand out a survey with two questions that may or may not even capture what desire feels like for a woman, Ussher conducted ninety-minute interviews asking college women, straight and lesbian, to describe in detail their experiences of desire. This kind of qualitative information gathering captures the nuances that the big demographic surveys can't. The women were asked open-ended questions about their experiences of desire, what it meant to them, and what other feelings came up along with desire. (Desire isn't always a pure stream of lust; if anxiety or self-consciousness is weaved in, the feeling is muddled.)

Ussher notes that "interpreting a feeling, thought or bodily change as 'sexual desire' is not a straightforward or automatic process. This is because the meaning of sexual experience is socially or discursively constructed, and thus sexual desire is partly a learnt phenomenon." The participants frequently reported nervousness as the first feeling to register, even before the spark of chemistry was fully realized. And lesbians additionally experienced confusion or panic at experiencing electricity toward another woman. These attendant feelings aren't typically considered when studies explore female desire. Anxiety has an effect on desire: it can enhance the excitement at low levels and totally obliterate it at higher levels—resulting not in a panic attack but blunted pleasure and numbness. This is a common occurrence that most of my clients don't fully understand until they've had some time to dissect what happens for them in the bedroom. If asked about their sex drive for a survey, surely they'd be more likely to report a low sex drive.

Another factor not commonly explored is how the roles women tend to play in the dance of attraction may affect the strength of that urge to fuck. In her interviews with straight women, Ussher aptly described this role as "doing girl," which is "knowingly taking up a position of archetypal femininity, of acquiescence and coquettishness." She also noted that straight women felt conscious that if they showed too much initiative they may appear too masculine and turn the guy off. The idea is that women behave passively because they want men to like them. They also reported wanting to avoid looking "easy" or like a "whore." Again, because they want men to like them. The women in the study actually were conscious of playing this role, indicating that there are still strong internalized forces against appearing sexually voracious. But what if they thought men would love it? Would women behave differently?

Enter the lesbians. These women didn't feel the same internal pressure to follow gender scripts. Ussher noticed that lesbian participants reported more fluidity in their roles. They reported a greater freedom to initiate, dominate, and switch again. Ussher wasn't able to say whether this fluidity led to a higher libido for lesbians. She didn't seem to want to create any easy generalizations. She simply made note of the many obstacles to lesbian desire, and her conclusion was that desire for women is indeed a complex process.

I think these roles of the wanting man and the desired woman, when fixed, are harmful to both genders. They don't give men the freedom to play the passive role, to enjoy her sexual authority. There is less flexibility; they don't get to shift power back and forth. My male clients tell me all the time that they wish women would be more sexually directive, expressive, and desirous. No need to "do girl." Thanks in part to LGBT studies and activism, I think we're finally on our way toward embracing a whole range of gender roles and a new narrative of freedom and agency for all.

Note:
A few of my favorite things

While exploring what sex was like before the Victorians told women we didn't have desire, I really got into finding ancient poems that celebrated sex. These are from a marvelous book published by Knopf called *Ancient Chinese Poems*.

The Untied Skirt
I hold my skirt, sash untied
And stand before the window with unpainted eyebrows

Silk clothes fly open so easily.
If my skirt opens, I'll blame the spring wind
(Zi Ye, 3rd century CE,)

Ancient Chinese poetry is abundant with expressions of women's desire. These poems were written in various political and social contexts in Chinese history, so the original meaning is probably different from my current interpretation. What's most important for the purpose of this book is how you interpret these poems now. As you read them, I ask you to consider how they interact with your worldview of sex, your body, and men's bodies. This one is about an unrequited desire:

Sleeping with One Pillow
You left in spring, leaving me with spring lust.
By summer that passion swells.
For whom do I lift my mosquito net?
When shall I have two pillows again?
(Zi Ye, 3rd century CE,)

I noticed a theme in Chinese poetry of an earthy, natural eroticism that weaves in the seasons and elements. It's always late at night and two lovers are sneaking into some orchard; words linger on a waist or a hair pin, red lips or jade fingers. The emotional longing of romantic love isn't necessarily present in these songs of desire. Shy or brazen, lonely or consummated, they are all about celebrating the experience of libido. Here her desire is aggressive:

Impatience
I want him so much
Want to crush him to me
To sit in his arms and nuzzle.
I'll call him. No, someone might hear.

The Women on My Couch

I'll drag him away. No, someone might see.
My eyes are fixed on him like a fatal foe
Until impatience murders me.
(Anonymous

This one is just a title, but frankly, enough said: "A Nun in Her Orchid Chamber Solitude Feels Lust Like a Monster". —Anonymous

This fragment reflects desire and enjoyment:

How could you resist a good man?
Who knows how to be gentle and sensuous?

These words don't give the impression that women were simply objects of pleasure for men or that women weren't sexual or that men's desire was greater. The next fragment of a poem seems endemic to the tone of their language about sex and body parts. (Note: "Jade stem" means penis.)

She softly shifts her willow waist
As he extends his jade stem fully,
Whispering desire for clouds and rain in the ear
Swearing oaths of mountain and sea in the pillow
(Anonymous)

Here is a description of a woman's body:

Creamy Breasts
Powdered, fragrant, sweat-soaked, they are round as pegs of a zither
Spring lust teases them into creamy melting, lingering rain, soft dough.
After her bath, where her man touches and plays with them
Magic flowers thicken into purple grapes
(Zhao Luanluan, 8th century)

Here is a little reflection on a woman's perception of her body:

Tangled Hair
Last night I didn't comb my hair
Like silk it tangles down my shoulders
And curls up on my knees
What part of me is not lovely?
(Zi Ye, 3rd century, p. 44)

The poetess Zi Ye, which means "Lady Midnight," was a professional singer and prominent poet during the Jing dynasty. I'm totally going to use that last line as an affirmation.

The ancient Chinese really linger on the amorous setting. Here is a fragment from a long poem describing a single traveler who comes upon a woman alone:

Fine scents hovered in the air
Rich screens and tapestries furnished it
And there in this room
A lady waited alone
Curvaceously beautiful, reclining on the bed
On the bed were laid
Exotic coverlets and sheets
A golden brazier breathed out scented smoke,
The curtains around the bed were lowered
(Sima Xiangru, 179–117 BCE)

The next poem is super ancient, from 600 BCE:

Stripping Off Clothes
If you miss me,
Strip your clothes and wade across the Zhen River to me

The Women on My Couch

If you do not miss me,
There are other men around
(Anonymous)

That's right, even way back, they knew about other fish in the sea.

Just to give you a sense of how political context has direct impact on libido, consider that, according to Jolan Cheng in the book *The Tao of Love and Sex*, the first Taoist writings on sexuality were developed when women shared equal status with men, just following a shift away from matriarchy to patriarchy. Thereafter, from the formation of the Han dynasty, a clear hierarchy was created and women became subservient, though, Cheng points out, people were still actively engaged in the harmonious sexual practices of Taoism. Gradually, women came to be distrusted, viewed as energetic vampires that depleted men. Women morphed into sexual enemies, described in antagonistic, even combative, terms.

History, of course, is not linear. There was a resurgence of the Tao in the Tang dynasty (AD 618–906), and then backward again, before foot binding was introduced around the tenth century. Foot binding started when imperial court dancers wore small shoes, followed by women of the aristocracy, who copied their fashion. Then, foot binding took on meaning. It became a status symbol for a woman who didn't have to work. The practice took hold as young women of lower classes viewed foot binding as a way to marry into wealthier families, again highlighting the role of economics and social meaning in what incites desire in humans. By the nineteenth century, 40 to 50 percent of women had bound feet, and it's thought that up to a billion Chinese women across the span of almost a thousand years crippled their feet in the name of sex appeal.

The Tao was corrupted and suppressed and perceived in a variety of ways throughout the lineage of Chinese dynasties, but there has been a modern worldwide resurgence.

Note:
Do guys *really* think about sex all day long?

How many times per day do you think about sex? How many times per day do you imagine the man in your life thinks about sex? Do you think there's a discrepancy?

A study from the *Journal of Sex Research* gave 283 college students a clicker to carry around all day. They were instructed to push the clicker each time they had a thought about sex, food, or sleep.

Get this, there was *no* significant gender difference in the frequency of thoughts about sex.

The young men, ages 18 to 25 (those we associate with the most extravagant sexual urges), did not think about sex the reputed every seven seconds. To be exact, these young men thought about sex between 1 and 388 times per day, a range so vast that it's hard to come up with an average. These hormone-raging, frothing young men did not even think about sex more frequently than food or sleep. And what about the women? The young women in the study thought of sex between 1 and 140 times per day, another range that doesn't allow any generalizations.

This study challenges the old myth that men think about sex all the time and that they think about it a great deal more than women do. The students who did the most "sex thought clicking" were also examined more closely to look for any patterns. If it's not about gender, what is associated with sexual thinking? The answer was very clear and actually did allow for a generalization: those who like sex and are comfortable with it think about it more often. This was true for both the men and the women in the study who scored in the high frequency range. This is an encouraging result for the purposes of sex therapy. If thoughts, attitudes, and behaviors around sexuality can be shifted from negative to affirmative, there may be hope for increasing desire in those who "just aren't feeling it."

Note:

"I have never deceived anyone, for I have never belonged to anyone. My independence was all my wealth: I have known no other happiness."

—Cora Pearl

Note:
A super-irritating study and its awesome takedown by an undergrad!

Evolutionary psychology has become popular in recent years, and its proclamations sound a lot like those of the medical papers I've seen in history books from the eighteenth century. Yet, questionnaires seem to keep confirming these ideas. One of the largest-scale studies on women's sex drive was published in 2007 by Richard Lippa of California State University. It involved a BBC Internet survey of 200,000 people from 53 nations. Lippa's results indicated that women across cultures have a lower sex drive than men. He used this finding to conclude that biology is the reason for the gender difference in sex drive, that libido is a matter of nature (though he does acknowledge the impact of culture). His findings indicated further that gender equality and economic development did not predict a better sex drive for women. This result seemed to go against everything that makes sense to me, so I scrutinized the survey to see whether there would be any clues as to why he got this result.

I discovered that Lippa's conclusion about the nature of a woman's sex drive was formed by asking only two questions. Although the survey included other questions assessing other aspects of sexuality, the libido component contained just two questions. Here they are: "I have a strong sex drive" and "It doesn't take much to get me sexually excited." Respondents chose an answer on a 7-point scale ranging from "agree" to "disagree." How the two of these statements were developed isn't mentioned in the study, but they fail to capture how female libido works in the first place.

It's widely accepted in sex therapy that women's desire often comes after being physically aroused (lubricated) and women sometimes even

170

reaches orgasm without much desire. Arousal can be ignited through foreplay, erotica, visual images, a hot guy who knows what he's doing, and so forth. She lubricates, and *then* she is interested in sex. Therefore, women aren't walking around sensing a strong sex drive, but when women are properly aroused, the desire for sex can be incredible. This is consistent with the ancient wisdom from China and India that value women's desire as different from men's but no less in strength. Wu Hsien, an ancient Taoist, advises: "The female belongs to Yin. Yin's peculiarity is that she is slow to be aroused but also slow to be satiated." The teachings of Tantra also instruct men on how to tap into a woman's fire through the right touches, usually involving breath and breast fondling before moving toward the clitoris, thus creating arousal first, and then desire.

However, even this concept of arousal before desire doesn't hold up in all situations. Women can certainly experience desire first or desire but no arousal or touch with no desire or arousal. Women can even experience arousal when the conditions are all wrong, such as in rape and sexual abuse. There is no singular story about how desire works, and that's hard for researchers to accept. There's no predictable pattern, which creates confusion about how a woman's desire operates, and therefore, our attempts at measurement are made on the basis of assumptions that don't reflect the way a woman's body actually works; thus, they yield erroneous results. The truth is that researchers of libido don't have definitive answers; some are still looking for the G-spot. What we do know, biologically speaking, is that a woman can have multiple orgasms and the clitoris is eight inches long (not in a straight line) and has more nerve endings than a penis.

Further, surveys like Lippa's capture only prevalence data: how often something is occurring; they don't address *why* it's occurring. The results sound good at face value, but just because the same answers repeat across studies doesn't make them truth, only popular—and they end up in magazines and Internet articles because they make for catchy headlines.

People often self-report on these types of questionnaires what they believe is expected. This reminds me of the studies mentioned in the book *Sex and the Citadel*, where Shereen El Feki reports on surveys conducted across the Middle East to see who is having sex before marriage. Most men said yes, and women said no. To get real answers, El Feki had to go to gynecologists' and therapists' offices. Another example is a study showing that Greek men report having the most sex (yes, of all humans on Earth! Researchers try to assess this from time to time). Truth or bravado? Hard to tell without a cultural analysis—which is what gets thrown wayside in evolutionary circles. Evolutionary theorists prefer instead to tell the genetic narrative.

Here is what Lippa makes of his findings in his own words:

> Because women are the "choosier" sex and because women often offer mating privileges to men in exchange for resources, protection, and commitment, it seems reasonable to hypothesize that sexual selection would endow women, on average, with less urgent sex drives that are more subject to rational control.

He goes on to state:

> Men's success at mating and reproduction tends to be more variable than women's and the highest levels of male success (defined here in terms of transmission of genes to future generations) may sometimes result from promiscuous sexual activity with multiple partners. Thus, sexual selection likely has led men, on average, to have stronger and more consistently "turned on" sex drives than women.

I can understand the allure of this simple biological logic. Sometimes I wish I chose an easier specialty so I could more often enjoy the gratification of therapy creating actual change. Treating low libido is difficult; often results are modest. However, just because a phenomenon appears ubiquitous doesn't mean it's a result of genetics. Libido is too sensitive, susceptible to many conditions: health, relationship, culture, mood, comfort level with being sexual, fear of being erotic. Further, when men present with low sex drive, it's also hard for them to get it rebooted. I think it's normal for libido to vacillate throughout the course of a day, month, and relationship—for women and men alike. At the time of this writing, my practice has more men with low sex drive than women.

The takedown: In 2011, Gina Silverstein, an undergraduate at Brown University, had an idea about why women are experiencing arousal issues. From listening to her friends, she knew that lots of young women were having trouble reaching orgasm or even getting turned on, and she noted that they often would say their mind was everywhere else but in the room. She had been taking a class on contemplative studies and had the idea of using the meditation technique of mindfulness to treat women's sexual problems. She approached a professor about creating a sex study in a lab dedicated to the effects of meditation. This undergrad student was able to rally on board several doctoral-level researchers.

The Brown study shoots a hole in the theories of those putting forth gender dictates. This research team, coming not from the sexology community but from the contemplative study community, finally addressed the question of why women report a less immediate and urgent drive toward sex. First, Silverstein determined that when women are turned on we're less likely to notice it than men are. More than one study has shown that a woman is actually wet and engorged, yet she is still saying she's not. This disconnect is even more pronounced in women with sexual dysfunction. This offers one explanation for Lippa's results. How can a woman respond accurately to his statement "It doesn't take much to get me sexually excited" if she doesn't know when she is sexually excited?

Silverstein and her team hypothesized there must be a psychological obstacle to women noticing their own horniness. From listening to her friends, she guessed the mental clatter of self-judgment about sex, including guilt, anxiety, embarrassment, and feelings of inadequacy, was the culprit.

To feel the sensations of sexual energy, we need focus, and when our mental awareness shifts to emotions or self-evaluation, we don't feel down there. By the way, this happens for men, too, and is the reason for most cases of erectile issues.

So, Gina Silverstein at Brown decided to do an experiment. She would use meditation as an intervention. Many studies tell us that meditation reduces anxiety and self-judgment and increases the ability to pay attention to the present. She wanted to see whether the gap between men's and women's arousal times would close if they meditated. She had a group of women meditate on a regular basis for 12 weeks and a control group of women who just took a music class. Silverstein also included a group of guys for comparison. At the end of the 12-week period, all the volunteers were shown a series of images, some sexy and some not, and were asked to report their level of arousal. As Silverstein predicted, the women who took the meditation classes had significantly shorter reaction times to the sexy images than did the women who took the music class. They also wound up with less anxiety, less self-criticism, and an improved ability to stay present.

I see this disconnect between mind and body in my practice all the time. I meet women who are full of ideas about sexual liberation, but when it comes to actual embodiment of those ideas, they don't always measure up and they can't figure out why. The Brown study is an important attempt to ask why rather than to accept survey results at face value. Although it was a smaller scale study than the 200,000-person megastudy conducted by Lippa, it was less superficial. Silverstein's results challenge this story that women's desire is lower by nature and suggest the answer may be, in fact, nurture.

So, what environmental reason would cause a pervasive pattern in women of blockage to the experience of libido? What are the deeper issues? There are the obvious answers, such as worrying about our weight or performance as a lover, and the less obvious, such as a primal embarrassment that seems to come out of nowhere. Finally, I think we should consider the history presented here, one that dates back to the nineteenth century, and how the extreme shame attached to being sexual may still be present each time we get in bed and may not allow us to fully delve into the sexual experience with unfettered abandon.

Note:
Wisdom from a psychologist and popular author who goes by the name of Starhawk

The symbolism of power—wealth, military force, physical prowess, and expressions of social status—is a constant presence in the United States. This can make domination in social, economic, and sexual relationships seem as if it's a normal part of humanity.

Starhawk, in her book *Dreaming the Dark: Magic, Sex, and Politics,* gives us a sense of where this dynamic came from. She traces the line of egalitarian and woman-centered spirituality that existed in Europe well past the rise of the Greek and Roman empires. She tells the history of the West's transition from feudalism to capitalism and how, at the same time, Paganism shifted to Christianity, which dramatically changed the social structure and thus sexuality.

Starhawk writes that pastoral Europeans formerly viewed sex as an egalitarian exchange of energy not at all separate from the life forces that were celebrated in nature. Of further note, she states that sado-masochistic activity didn't seem to be prevalent. She proposes that these power dynamics we've come to accept aren't natural but are learned. We've learned hierarchy in our families and our cultures. We experience it in our workplaces. Over time, the power-over dynamic became a part of European sexual behavior, and we haven't questioned it much since. In fact, it's lauded in sex therapy circles.

Note:
Excerpt from my interview with orgasm guru Kim Anami

I interviewed Kim and asked whether she thought a woman's desire for sex could be as strong as a man's. She said:

> As, or stronger. Women have no refractory periods in sex! That ought to tell you something. Yes, it's naturally stronger, but as I said, we've—men and women—been conditioned to think otherwise. A sexually voracious woman is a fearsome thing.

That's why there are so many myths and stories about her. When a woman truly owns her sexuality, she steps into a deep power and confidence she never knew she had. She becomes unshakeable. The world is her oyster.

I also asked her if a woman's libido ignited differently than a man's, and she replied:

There is an old Taoist adage that, sexually speaking, men are like fire: quick to ignite and quick to extinguish. Women are like water: slow to boil but they keep on boiling. It isn't true that women are stimulated more by emotions than men. We've all been conditioned to believe that though. Men and women need emotional and physical stimulation equally. However, we've been conditioned to believe that women are more "emotional" and men more "physical." It's only true to the extent that we've internalized it.

I concur with her observations. I see a lot of distress between couples when his desire is strong and immediate and she feels pressure that she can't match it. Further, neither understand how to incite her desire.

Note:
The sexual intimacy paradox

Cut from the Laura chapter: In graduate school, as I was trying to figure out why so many people had good relationships but bad sex, I came across some startling research by Charles Lobitz and Gretchen Lobitz (1996), who found that marital therapy aimed at increasing emotional intimacy was actually correlated with a decline in sexual desire. Further, studies demonstrated that techniques aimed to improve communication were at times associated with an *increase* in sexual problems. It seemed as if a good relationship was a precursor to bad sex. Lobitz and Lobitz dubbed this the "sexual intimacy paradox."

The authors also reported what actually incites lust: distance, mystery, novelty, danger, and power differences. This sounded like a poor prognosis for the relationship ideals of modern monogamy. Should Laura be scared that she loved to throw on her flannel jammie pants, watch HBO, and snuggle at night or that Brian folds laundry and she takes out the trash? Or that domestic matters were negotiated in weekly family meetings? Is this really a dangerous threat to marriages? As I thought this through, I became dubious, not about monogamy or the egalitarian relationship but about the purported "comfortable couples" described in the research. This word, "comfortable," seemed to me a red flag. I noticed a flaw in the face value of this sexual intimacy paradox.

I don't think emotional intimacy destroys passion, as the sexual intimacy paradox may lead us to believe. The truth is that humans are neurologically wired for intimacy. We *need* it. However, in a monogamous relationship, there isn't much distance or mystery—particularly if you live together.

We think we need mystery, danger, and novelty, but isn't this putting even more of a burden on our partner? How can the person who's there to wipe your nose when you're sick also be a source of danger? How can the person who holds you each night also amuse with constant novelty?

Sexual desire requires difference. There is room for two personalities, two solid individuals. That same friction that can be annoying can also be a source of passion when managed right. The key is to learn how to hold on to yourself. The process of joining two lives will challenge your sense of self on a regular basis. When the idiosyncrasies of each partner collide, there needs to be a balancing act of holding your ground and respecting the other as a free individual—*at the same time.*

Further, it's easy to blame egalitarian relationships for being as hot as a winter day in Providence. But in truth, the problem that plagues most couples isn't the equal division of responsibilities but the grossly unsexy behaviors most people do in relationships: pleasing, ingratiating, controlling, or being judgmental, selfish, lazy, and other forms of general assholery. Many studies falsely compare egalitarian relationships with

hierarchical ones—as if these are the only two options. As if these neu-
tralized gender roles lauded by the likes of Brian and Laura and their
cohorts are upending some natural order. I have clients tell me all the
time that they prefer traditional gender roles. It's sexier. But I guarantee
that Brian and Laura's respectful and democratic-communication-lov-
ing, boundary-negotiating friends are having some pretty wild sex. And
this crowd is not the first in human history to explore homosexuality,
group sex, or sex outside one's relationship, as evidenced by the *Kama
Sutra*, originally composed four hundred years before Christ.

The fallacy I see in the sexual intimacy paradox lies in the label
"comfortable." A deeper look at the couples in the Lobitz study might
reveal pairs that are merged yet empty, content yet desperate. Lobitz and
Lobitz mention that the way out of the comfortable couple syndrome
is to push past your comfort zone, to incorporate new ways of playing
with distance, novelty, danger, and power differences. To do this requires
letting go of fear-based constrictions and allowing yourself to become
more sexually open and expansive. Is that with a threesome—or by
looking into each other's eyes? For each couple, it's unique.

Art Aron, a professor at Stony Brook University who developed the
"self-expansion theory" of attraction, says that our differences, not our
similarities, stimulate excitement in the initial stages of a relationship.
We like how meeting someone new introduces us to new activities,
new places, and new ways of thinking about the world. When the
learning process stagnates, passion withers along with it. I asked a friend
who had been married almost thirty years how he stays attracted to his
wife. He said, "I keep falling in love, over and over—with other things."
He said his creative endeavors sate his need for excitement and passion,
which he brings back to the marriage. Sounds worth the effort—at the
very least I'd be an old person with a lot of hobbies. The idea to take
away here is, the more you expand yourself, the more you expand your
partner. The result is that the novelty, mystery, and possibly even danger
of bringing fresh interests into the relationship keep it simmering.

Note:
Random experience

Once in Cairo, I ventured to what I thought would be an evening of dinner and dance, which was actually a strip club—maybe even a sex club. My companion, an elderly woman who had been traveling alone, and I were served a mediocre dinner, and while we ate, a series of women in tight dresses danced across the stage. Then, a woman appeared clad in a long, flowing Islamic dress, with a headscarf and another scarf covering her mouth and nose. Only her eyes were visible. She glided across the stage, moving her body so that you would catch glimpses of it pressing out against the fabric, and then lose them again in the movement. I was like, *Holy shit, I'm in a strip club watching a woman dance in a burka.* Her hands, unhidden, turned delicately, her fingers slowly undulating through the air. She carefully gazed at you and then away. She was the most captivating dancer, though she never removed an article of clothing. She engaged the mystery of the body, inciting desire to see beneath her cloak. I looked around the room and noticed the men were really into her.

Note:

Cutline: There's this fin sticking up from under the sheets and it's swimming toward me, like Jaws. She rolled her eyes at me, as if looking for some feminine commiseration at the menacing morning erection.

Note:

Cut from Lilu chapter: We're all familiar with that famed era of repression, the Victorian age. For my eighth-grade dance, my mom dressed me as an actual Victorian. She took me to the mall to shop for a dress. We passed through the aisles of the department store junior section party dresses, and I started fondling various sequined dresses. My mother promptly told me she wasn't buying any of those dresses.

So, I followed her around in some dissociated state of disappointment, not even looking anymore because I knew not to push for what I wanted. My mother was determined to dress me. She somehow found a long peach skirt with a big ruffle at the bottom and a cream-colored turtleneck sweater with lace embellishments along the décolletage—a feature that, she pointed out, was quite lovely. She tried in vain to sell me on this outfit for my dance. I told her I hated it. She bought the items and we went home.

Sullen, I allowed her to do my hair. And, accordingly, she coiffed a bun atop my head and of course allowed no makeup. Seriously proud of her chaste-looking little lady, she dropped me, in full Victorian regalia, off in front of my best friend Maria's house. Her mistake was that she didn't come inside.

Maria's was an Italian family in a blue-collar neighborhood in Pittsburgh. I walked in the front door and Maria's family all turned to stare. The response: "Oh my Gawwwd! What the hell do you have on?" And that was her mom. Then, roars of laughter as I stood haplessly in my itchy lace and wool nineteenth-century frock.

Minutes later I was teasing my bangs, applying blue eyeliner, and slipping into an age-inappropriate sexy dress—I think it was Maria's mother's.

Note:
A final reason to be sexual

I would be remiss if I didn't provide, at a minimum, some acknowledgment of the physiological aspects of sex. This isn't a book to explain the mechanics of the body, hormones, or the sexual response system and its potential ailments; that's all been written about comprehensively elsewhere. Here, I simply comment on how health relates to desire.

I once viewed intimacy as an expression of something primarily interpersonal. It was about passion or love or play. I never considered it personal, essential to my overall well-being. Learning what intercourse actually provided for my body gave me a whole new frame for the purpose of sex. So, if you've ever wondered why you should care about increasing your libido, perhaps this will provide a new perspective. There is a great deal of research out there to support the health benefits of sex, and here are the highlights:

- *Boosts the immune system:*
  Having sex once or twice per week raises your immunoglobulin levels, helping to protect you from colds and other infections.
- *Strengthens the heart:*
  Sex improves cardiovascular health and circulation. Studies show that sex decreases the risk of heart attack and stroke, and—this part fascinates me the most—sex is particularly healthful when the tone is loving.
- *Reduces stress:*
  Sex lowers blood pressure and releases hormones that relax the body and promote a sense of mental well-being. Orgasms help flush out cortisol, the stress hormone.
- *Reduces pain:*
  Sex releases endorphins and the powerful hormone oxytocin, both of which reduce pain. Studies report improvement for migraines, PMS, and arthritis.
- *Improves insomnia:*
  The hormone oxytocin promotes sleep.
- *Makes you look younger:*
  Studies show that the skin appears younger and more firm with more sex.

For Taoists, sex is medicine. Two thousand years ago, the Chinese didn't view sex as dirty or immoral but as nourishing and replenishing. Its tenor was wholesome, natural. From this perspective, sex isn't some act you have to perform to keep a rapacious man satisfied. These health benefits are for you.

This idea is important to consider when contemplating the nature of a woman's desire. If women were designed to have sex only during some short-lived "romantic phase," then why would ongoing sex have so many health implications? If you look at the advantages, it seems sex should be a part of a healthy lifestyle at any age. It aids in keeping systems regulated: immune, circulatory, and endocrine. Sex is like a wellness benefit; your insurance should give you incentive points for it.

The Women on My Couch

Taoism, in short, posits that the flow of energy is the source of life. Energy, or *chi*, can sound like some esoteric concept to Westerners but in fact has been a recognized part of health in many cultures. Sex, Taoist style, is all about the joining of essences. Yin and Yang were thought to be complementary forces and of equal value. The emphasis was on the exchange of essences to create harmony for the health of both genders and peace in society at large.

Living an erotic lifestyle was important to the Taoists. For them, eroticism was an art and a skill that could be taught. They even had "love masters." Many modern women are averse to learning a system of techniques, viewing it as mechanical. I used to think the same way. I thought that having to use techniques meant that you were trying too hard or that you were doing something that wasn't spontaneous and, therefore, somehow not real passion. It took me a long time to summon the patience to actually look at the intercourse position list (though positions do have some awesome names, like *A Singing Monkey Holding a Tree, Two Fishes Side-by-Side,* and *Phoenix Holding Her Chicken*).

In his popular book, *The Tao of Love and Sex,* Jolan Chang highlights how to touch.

> While making love, neither of you should stop touching each other with your hands, until you are both tired and ready to sleep....A woman's clitoris and breasts are usually her most sensitive spots. But do not touch her here immediately: caress her hands and kiss her first. A woman is also sensitive on or near her spinal column from head to hips and thighs. These points vary from woman to woman but the most popular ones are the ears, the back of the neck and around the waist, especially in the back. The inside of the thighs are also very sensitive. Her abdomen is often caressed by your abdomen—one of the great joys of loving.

I assure you these lessons in love are not as rigid as, say, a game of Twister: "Right hand on red, left hand on boob." The Taoists were masters of seduction with superlative display: silk robes, perfumed curtains, and the dim lighting of red lanterns. They also used explicit artwork as part of their seduction process, images that have none of the pejorative connotations of today's visual stimulation.

Note:

I have taken off my robe—
Must I put it on again?
I have washed my feet—
Must I soil them again?
My lover thrust his hand through the latch
And my heart began to pound for him
I arose to open for my lover
And my hands dripped with myrrh,
My fingers with flowing myrrh
Upon the handles of the bolt
I opened for my lover
But my lover had left; he was gone
My heart sank at his departure.
I looked for him but did not find him
Oh, daughters of Jerusalem, I charge you—
If you find my lover
Tell him I am faint with love.
(Song of Solomon, Chapter 5, Holy Bible)

Buddhahood is obtained from bliss—
And apart from women
There will not be bliss.
(Candamaharosana)

An orgasm a day keeps the doctor away.
(Mae West)

The Women on My Couch

How beautiful you are and how pleasing
O love with your delights!
Your stature is like that of the palm,
And your breasts like clusters of fruit
I will climb the palm tree and I will take hold of its fruit
May your breasts be like clusters of the vine,
The fragrance of your breath like apples
And your mouth like the best wine
(Song of Songs, 7:6–9, Holy Bible)

Before lowering the perfumed curtain to express her love,
She knits her eyebrows, worried that the night is too short.
She urges the young lover to go to bed
First, so as to warm-up the mandarin-duck quilt
A moment later she puts down her unfinished needlework
And removes her silk skirt, to indulge in passion
Without end.
(Lui Yung, 990–1050)

My vulva, the horn, The Boat of Heaven is full of
eagerness like the young moon
Who will plow my vulva? Who will plow my high field?
Who will plow my wet ground?
Great Lady, the King will plow your vulva.
Then plow my vulva, man of my heart!
...at the Kings lap stood the rising cedar.
Plants grew high by their side. Gardens flourished luxuriantly.
(The Hymns of Innana, recorded on ancient Sumerian stone tablets)

With his venom
Irresistible
And bittersweet
That loosener
Of limbs, Love

Reptile like
Strikes me down

(Sappho,
ancient Greece)

We move beyond speech
Our bodies move past all the controls we have learned.
We cry out in ecstasy, in feeling…
To touch another is to express love: there is no idea apart
from feeling, and no feeling that does not ring through our
bodies and our souls at once.
This is Eros. Our own wholeness. Not the sensation of
pleasure alone, nor the idea of love alone, but the whole
experience of human love. The whole of human
experience exists in this love. Here is the capacity for speech and
meaning, for culture, for memory, for imagination…
(Susan Griffin)

She sits naked on a rock
A few yards out in the water
He stands on the shore
Also naked, picking blueberries.

She calls. He turns.
She opens her legs
Showing him
Her great beauty
(fragment from *The Last Gods* by Galway Kinnell)
(He's not ancient, by the way. This is just one of my favorite poems.)

I honor those who reverence my power but lay low of all
those whose thoughts toward me are proud.
(Aphrodite in Euripides, *Hippolytus*)

Acknowledgments

I'd like to thank David Rensin, co-author of *The Men on My Couch*, who spent time reading the early drafts that were dense and full of error, patiently and lovingly offering detailed direction and critique, all while he was busy with his own, soon to be best-selling, writing project. Even though I wanted to branch out on my own, I can't deny the role his guidance played in me finding my own voice. I am grateful for his mentorship and friendship. Thank you also, to his talented son, Emmett Rensin, magazine writer and playwright, who has worked on editing bits of my book and articles. I feel certain he'll be famous one day and I can boast that he once edited my work.

I'd like to thank my husband, Francis Engler for his unwavering support. Thank you for reading, offering feedback and believing in me when I felt doubtful about my ability to write. He also accompanied me to Greece to do the Minoan research—but he can thank me for that. I also want to thank Mark and Paul Engler, both authors, whom provided advice and good conversations about writing. And I'd like to thank the rest of the extended Engler clan for reading my material and always showing interest and curiosity—even when such topics aren't the most comfortable to share with family over a Thanksgiving dinner.

I'd also like to thank Naomi Long and Christina Yeager at The Artful Editor, Susannah Martin and Leslie Cook for your careful edits. I'd also like to thank Amy Reichenbach, Karen Bethzabe, Sue Shrader and my dear parents, Bob and Irene Dunn.

Suggested Readings

Acevedo, B., & Aron, A. (2009). Does a long-term relationship kill romantic love? *Review of General Psychology, 13*(1), 59–65.

Aries, P., & Bejin, A. (1982). *Western sexuality*. Oxford, England: Basil Blackwell.

Aron, A., Norman, C. C., Aron, E. N., McKenna, C., & Heyman, R. E. (2000). Couples' shared participation in novel and arousing activities and experienced relationship quality. *Journal of Personality and Social Psychology, 78*(2), 273–284.

Arroba, A. (2001). *New view of women's sexuality: The case of Costa Rica*. Place TK: Haworth Press.

Barnstone, T., & Ping, C. (2007). *Chinese erotic poems*. New York, NY: Everyman's Library Pocket Poets.

Basson, R. (2001). Using a different model for female sexual response to address women's problematic low sexual desire. *Journal of Sex & Marital Therapy, 27*, 395–403.

Blatchford, W. (1983) *Grande Horizontal*. Stein and Day. New York.

Bergner, D. (2013). *What do women want?* New York, NY: HarperCollins.

Brooks, G. (1995). *Nine parts of desire*. New York, NY: Anchor Books.

Cahill, T. (2003). *Sailing the wine-dark sea: Why the Greeks matter*. New York, NY: Anchor Books.

Chang, J. (1997). *The Tao of love and sex*. New York, NY: Penguin.

Charlton, R., & Yalom, I. (1997). *Treating sexual disorders*. San Francisco, CA: Jossey-Bass.

Chia, M., & Abrams, R. (2005). *The multi-orgasmic woman*. Emmaus, PA: Rodale.

Clarke, J. (1998). *Looking at lovemaking*. Berkeley: University of California Press.

Corbin, A. (1990). *Women for hire*. Cambridge, MA: Harvard University Press.

Doidge, N. (2007). *The brain that changes itself*. London, England: Penguin.

Dove, N., & Weiderman, M. (2000). Cognitive distraction and women's sexual functioning. *Journal of Sex & Marital Therapy, 26*, 67–78.

Everaerd, W., & Laan, E. (1995). Desire for passion: Energetics of sexual response. *Journal of Sex & Marital Therapy, 27*, 247–257.

Feki, S. (2013). *Sex and the citadel*. New York, NY: Pantheon Books.

Fitton, G. (2002). *Minoans*. London, England: British Museum Press.

Fontes, L. (2001). The new view and Latina sexualities: *Pero no soy una maquina!* Place TK: Haworth Press.

Frankl, V. (1995). *Man's search for meaning*. New York, NY: Washington Square Press.

Friday, N. (1998). *My secret garden*. New York, NY: Pocket Books.

Gere, C. (2009). *Knossos and the prophets of modernism*. Chicago, IL: University of Chicago Press.

Greeff, A., & Malherbe, H. (2001). Intimacy and marital satisfaction in spouses. *Journal of Sex & Marital Therapy, 27*, 225–263.

Griffin, S. (2001). *The book of the courtesans*. New York, NY: Broadway Books.

Guay, A. (2001). Decreased testosterone in regularly menstruating women with decreased libido: A clinical observation. *Journal of Sex & Marital Therapy, 27*(5), 513–519.

Hamilakis, Y. (2010). *Labyrinth revisited*. Oxford, England: Oxbow Books.

Hawkes, J. (1910). *Dawn of the gods*. New York, NY: Random House.

Hawton, K. (1985). *Sex therapy: A practical guide*. New York, NY: Oxford University Press.

Heiman, J. R., & Meston, C. M. (1997). Empirically validated treatment for sexual dysfunction. *Annual Review of Sex Research, 8,* 148–194.

Hickman, K. (2003). Courtesans: Money, Sex and Fame in the 19th Century. William Morrow

Holden, W. (1950) *The Pearl from Plymouth: Eliza Emma Crouch, alias Cora Pearl.*. The British Technical and General Press.

Horney, K. (1937). *The neurotic personality of our time.* New York, NY: W. W. Norton.

Horney, K. (1945). *Our inner conflicts.* New York, NY: W. W. Norton.

Kaplan, H. S. (1974). *The new sex therapy.* New York, NY: Brunner/Mazel.

Kaplan, H. S. (1977). Hypoactive sexual desire. *Journal of Sex & Marital Therapy, 3,* 3–9.

Kaplan, H. S. (1995). *The sexual desire disorders.* New York, NY: Brunner/Mazel.

Klein, M. (1997). Disorders of desire. In R. Charlton (Ed.), *Treating sexual disorders* (pp. 201–236). San Francisco, CA: Jossey-Bass.

Lippa, R. (2007). Sex differences in sex drive, sociosexuality, and height across 53 nations: Testing evolutionary and social structural theories. *Archives of Sexual Behavior, 38*(5), 631–651.

Lobitz, C., & Lobitz, J. (1996). Resolving the sexual intimacy paradox: A developmental model for the treatment of sexual desire disorders. *Journal of Sex & Marital Therapy, 22,* 71–83.

MacPhee, D., & Johnson, S. (1995). Low sexual desire in women: The effects of marital therapy. *Journal of Sex & Marital Therapy, 21,* 159–181.

Marinatos, N. (1984). *Art and religion in Thera: Reconstructing a Bronze Age society.* Athens, Greece: D. & I. Mathioulakis.

Masters, W. H., & Johnson, V. (1970). *Human sexual inadequacy.* Boston, MA: Little, Brown.

McCabe, M. (2001). Evaluation of a cognitive behavioral therapy program for people with a sexual dysfunction. *Journal of Sex & Marital Therapy, 27*(3), 259–271.

McCarthy, B. (1997). Strategies and techniques for revitalizing a nonsexual marriage. *Journal of Sex & Marital Therapy, 23*, 231–240.

McCarthy, B. (1999). Relapse prevention strategies and techniques for inhibited sexual desire. *Journal of Sex & Marital Therapy, 25*, 297–303.

Mendus, S., & Rendall, J. (1989). *Sexuality and subordination.* London, England: Routledge.

Miller, K. A. (2008). Sarah Water's *Fingersmith*: Leaving women's fingerprints on Victorian pornography. *Nineteenth-Century Gender Studies Journal*, 4.1. Retrieved from http://www.ncgsjournal.com/issue41/miller.htm

Ministry of Culture Archaeological Receipts Fund. (2004). *The ring of Minos.* Athens, Greece: Archaeological Fund.

Moore, T. (1998). *The soul of sex.* New York, NY: HarperCollins.

Myers, D. (1999). *Social psychology.* Boston, MA: McGraw-Hill.

Neruda, P. (1952). *The captain's verses.* New York, NY: New Directions.

Pasahow, C. (2003). *Sexy encounters.* Place TK: Adams Media.

Pearl, C. (2012). *The memoirs of Cora Pearl: The English beauty of the French empire...* London, England: Nabu Public. (Original work published 1890)

Pridal, C., & LoPiccolo, J. (2000). Multielement treatment of desire disorders: Integration of cognitive, behavioral, and systemic therapy. In S. Leiblum & R. Rosen (Eds.), *Principles and practice of sex therapy* (pp. 00–00). New York, NY: Guilford Press.

Resnik, S. (1997). *The pleasure zone.* Berkeley, CA: Canari Press.

Resnik, S. (2004). Somatic-experiential sex therapy: A body-centered Gestalt approach to sexual concerns. *Gestalt Review, 8*(1), 40–64.

Richardson, D. (2003). *The heart of Tantric sex.* Place TK: O Books.

Royalle, C. (2004). *How to tell a naked man what to do.* New York, NY: Simon & Schuster.

Safir, M. (2001). *An Israeli sex therapist considers a new view of women's sexual problems.* Place TK: Haworth Press.

Sawer, D., & Durlak, J. (1997). A field trial of the effectiveness of behavioral treatment for sexual dysfunctions. *Journal of Sex & Marital Therapy, 23*, 87–95.

Schnarch, D. (1991). *Constructing the sexual crucible*. New York, NY: W. W. Norton.

Schnarch, D. (1997). *Passionate marriage: Keeping love and intimacy alive in committed relationships*. New York, NY: W. W. Norton.

Schnarch, D. (2000). Desire problems: A systemic perspective. In S. Leiblum & R. Rosen (Eds.), *Principles and practice of sex therapy* (pp. 17–56). New York, NY: Guilford Press.

Schwartz, L. (2001). Family systems discourse: Conversations with clients concerning the impact of family legacies on sexual desire. *Journal of Sex & Marital Therapy, 27*, 603–606.

Silverstein, R. G., Brown, A.-C. H., Roth, H. D., & Britton, W. B. (2011). Effects of mindfulness training on body awareness to sexual stimuli: Implications for female sexual dysfunction. *Psychosomatic Medicine, 73*, 1–9.

Smith, E. E. (2013). There's no such thing as everlasting love (according to science). *The Atlantic*. Retrieved from http://www.theatlantic.com/sexes/archive/2013/01/theres-no-such-thing-as-everlasting-love-according-to-science/267199/

Smith, N. (2008). *Ancient philosophy*. Malden, MA: Blackwell.

Smith, W. (1985). *Second empire and commune: France 1848–1871*. London, England: Longman Group.

Starhawk. (1982). *Dreaming the dark*. Boston, MA: Beacon Press.

Stop Porn Culture. (2011). Facts and figures. Retrieved from http://stoppornculture.org/about/about-the-issue/facts-and-figures-2/

Ussher, J. (2005). The meaning of sexual desire: Experiences of heterosexual and lesbian girls. *Feminism & Psychology, 15*(1), 27–32.

Vasilakis, A. (2000). *Herakleion Archaeological Museum*. Place TK: Adam Editions.

Versluis, A. (2008). *The secret history of Western sexual mysticism*. Rochester, NY: Destiny Books.

Villacorta, N. (2011, November 10). Contemplating to climax: Meditation relieves sex woes. *Brown Daily Herald*.

Vohra, S. (2001). *New view of women's sexuality: The case of India*. Place TK: Haworth Press.

Warnock, J. (2002). Female hypoactive sexual desire disorder. Epidemiology, diagnosis and treatment. *CNS Drugs, 16*, 745–753.

Yalom, I. (1980). *Existential psychotherapy*. New York, NY: Basic Books.

Made in the USA
Coppell, TX
21 November 2019